The Flavorful Plant-Based Cookbook for Beginners

1800+ Days of Exciting and Mouthwatering Recipes to Spice Up Your Plant-Based Meals and Create a Healthier Lifestyle. Incl. 30 Days Meal Plan

Richard S. Stone

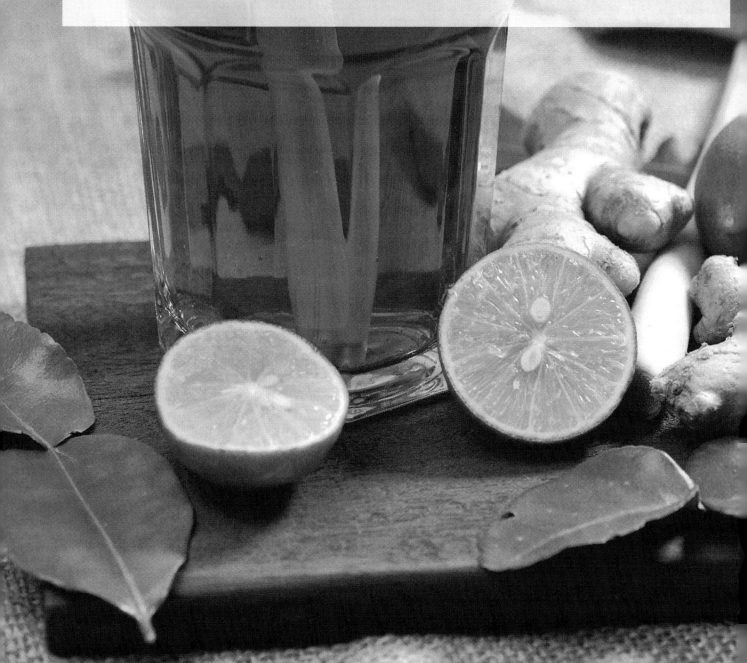

Copyright© 2024 By Richard S. Stone
All rights reserved worldwide.

No part of this book may be reproduced or transmitted in any form or by any means, electronic or mechanical, including photo- copying, recording or by any information storage and retrieval system, without written permission from the publisher, except for the inclusion of brief quotations in a review.

Warning-Disclaimer

The purpose of this book is to educate and entertain. The author or publisher does not guarantee that anyone following the techniques, suggestions, tips, ideas, or strategies will become successful. The author and publisher shall have neither liability or responsibility to anyone with respect to any loss or damage caused, or alleged to be caused, directly or indirectly by the information contained in this book.

Table of Contents

Introduction 01

Chapter 1 Understanding Plant-Based Diet 03

Chapter 2 Breakfasts 10

Chapter 3 Basics 20

Chapter 4 Beans and Grains 27

Chapter 5 Desserts 36

Chapter 6 Vegetables and Sides 45

Chapter 7 Snacks and Appetizers 55

Chapter 8 Salads 66

Chapter 9 Stews and Soups 76

Chapter 10 Staples, Sauces, Dips, and Dressings 88

Appendix 1: Measurement Conversion Chart 98

Appendix 2: The Dirty Dozen and Clean Fifteen 99

Appendix 3: Recipe Index 100

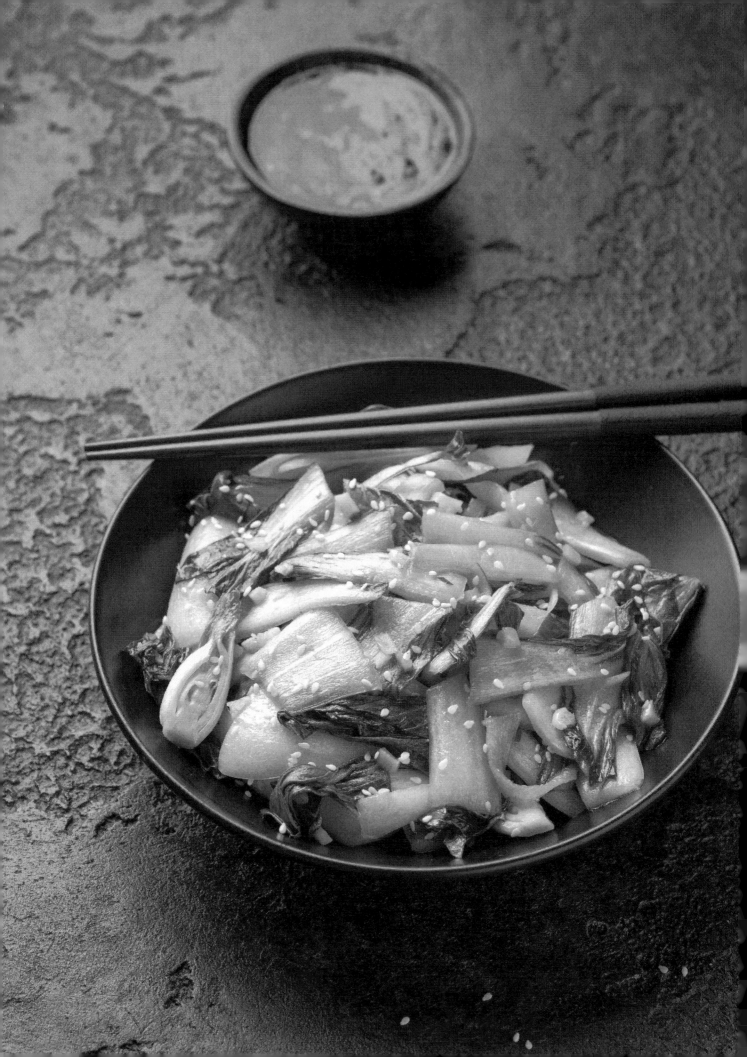

Introduction

Discover a culinary odyssey that transcends boundaries, where vibrant colors, tantalizing flavors, and boundless creativity converge on the pages of our plant-based diet cookbook. Welcome to a gastronomic wonderland where plants take center stage, showcasing their extraordinary potential to nourish both body and soul. In this culinary voyage, we embark on a transformative journey, unearthing the secrets of nature's bountiful pantry and presenting them to you in a collection of delectable recipes that will redefine your perception of what a plant-based diet can be.

Prepare to be enchanted as we unlock the doors to a world brimming with diversity, where the humble vegetable becomes a culinary superstar, the mighty legume unveils its hidden powers, and the delicate herbs and spices add a touch of magic to each dish. Our cookbook is a testament to the boundless possibilities that arise when we embrace the abundant gifts of the earth and celebrate the power of mindful eating.

But this cookbook is not just about nourishment—it's a gateway to a new way of living. As you explore its pages, you'll find more than just recipes; you'll encounter a harmonious fusion of art and science, as we dive into the nutritional benefits and healing properties of each ingredient. We'll empower you with knowledge, equipping you to make informed choices about your well-being, while never compromising on taste or satisfaction.

Whether you're a seasoned vegan seeking fresh inspiration or a curious food enthusiast eager to explore the vibrant world of plant-based cuisine, this cookbook will become your trusted companion. From breakfast delights that greet each day with a burst of energy, to soul-warming soups that comfort and nourish, to stunning main courses that will impress even the most skeptical of palates, our collection embraces the full spectrum of flavors and textures, ensuring every meal is a celebration of life.

So, embark on this culinary voyage with us, and let the pages of our plant-based diet cookbook guide you to a world of vibrant flavors, wholesome ingredients, and a renewed connection to the earth. Together, let's redefine the possibilities of food and embrace a lifestyle that not only nurtures our bodies but also leaves a positive impact on the world we share. Get ready to savor the extraordinary and embark on a journey where the extraordinary begins on your plate.

As the author of this plant-based diet cookbook, let me take you on a personal journey that ignited my passion for this transformative way of eating and led me to share my experiences with the world.

Several years ago, I found myself caught in the whirlwind of a fast-paced, stress-filled lifestyle. My days were consumed by endless to-do lists, and my body paid the price for neglecting its needs. I constantly felt drained, lacking the vitality and zest for life that I once possessed. It was a wake-up call that urged me to reevaluate my priorities and seek a healthier, more sustainable path.

In my quest for change, I stumbled upon the concept of a plant-based diet—an approach that emphasizes whole, unprocessed foods derived from nature's vibrant palette. Intrigued by its promises of vitality and well-being, I decided to embark on this journey, embracing the abundant array of fruits, vegetables, legumes, and grains that nature provided.

As I transitioned to a plant-based lifestyle, I was amazed at the immediate positive impact it had on my well-being. Energy flooded back into my days, replacing fatigue with vigor. My skin glowed with newfound radiance, and the excess weight I had carried for years effortlessly melted away. But the physical transformations were just the beginning.

With each plant-based meal, I felt a renewed sense of connection—to the Earth, to the animals we share it with, and to myself. I discovered that food could be a source of joy and nourishment, a way to express my creativity in the kitchen, and a means to make a positive difference in the world. The plant-based diet became not just a lifestyle but a philosophy—an invitation to live in harmony with nature and honor the interconnectedness of all living beings.

Inspired by my own transformation and fueled by a desire to share this profound experience, I decided to write this cookbook. It became my mission to demystify plant-based cooking, to celebrate the remarkable flavors and textures that plant-based ingredients offer, and to guide others on their own path to wellness.

Within the pages of this cookbook, you'll find not only a collection of mouthwatering recipes but also a reflection of my own culinary adventures and discoveries. It's a testament to the endless possibilities of plant-based cuisine, a gateway to a world where food becomes a celebration of life and a catalyst for positive change.

Through this cookbook, I hope to inspire you to embark on your own journey—a journey that nourishes not only your body but also your spirit. May it empower you to make conscious choices, embrace the vibrant tapestry of plant-based ingredients, and savor the extraordinary flavors that nature so generously provides.

Together, let us create a future where our plates are not only a source of sustenance but also a testament to our commitment to a more compassionate and sustainable world. Welcome to a culinary adventure that will nourish, delight, and awaken your senses—a journey where the extraordinary begins on your plate.

Chapter 1 Understanding Plant-Based Diet

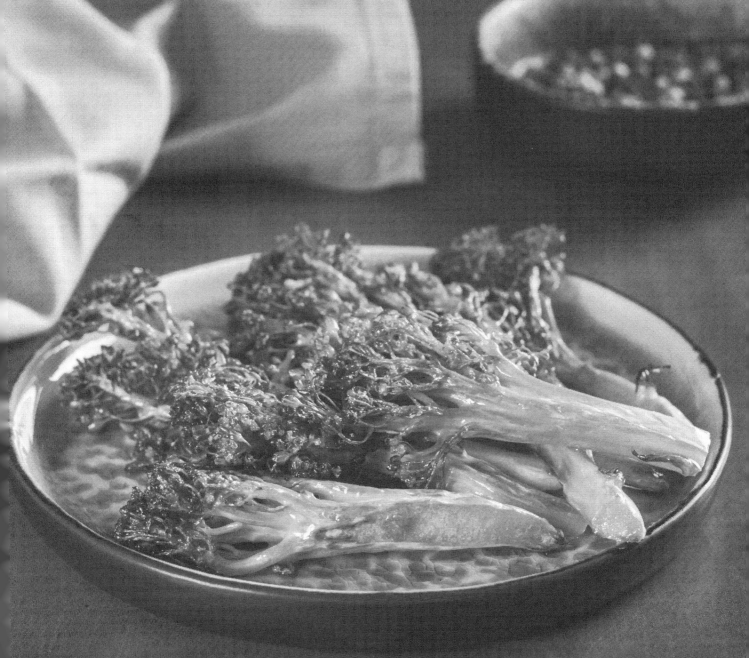

A plant-based diet is a way of eating that focuses on whole, minimally processed foods derived from plants. This means that the majority of your meals will consist of fruits, vegetables, whole grains, legumes, nuts, and seeds.

A plant-based diet has numerous health benefits, including reducing the risk of heart disease, diabetes, and certain types of cancer. It is also beneficial for weight management, as plant-based foods tend to be lower in calories and higher in fiber than animal-based foods.

In addition to the health benefits, a plant-based diet is also more sustainable for the environment, as it requires fewer resources to produce plant-based foods compared to animal-based foods.

Making the transition to a plant-based diet can be challenging at first, but there are many resources available to help you get started. You can begin by gradually incorporating more plant-based meals into your diet and experimenting with different recipes and ingredients. Over time, you may find that you prefer the taste and feel better on a plant-based diet.

Benefits of Plant-Based Diet

A plant-based diet has numerous benefits for both your health and the environment. Here are some of the key benefits:

1. Lower risk of chronic diseases: A plant-based diet has been linked to a lower risk of chronic diseases such as heart disease, diabetes, and certain types of cancer. This is because plant-based foods are typically lower in saturated fat and higher in fiber, vitamins, minerals, and antioxidants.

2. Better weight management: Plant-based foods tend to be lower in calories and higher in fiber than animal-based foods, making them a great choice for weight management. Studies have shown that people who follow a plant-based diet tend to have a lower body mass index (BMI) and are less likely to be overweight or obese.

3. Improved gut health: Plant-based foods are rich in fiber, which helps to promote healthy digestion and prevent constipation. Fiber also feeds the beneficial bacteria in your gut, which can improve overall gut health and reduce the risk of certain diseases.

4. Reduced inflammation: Many plant-based foods are rich in anti-inflammatory compounds, which can help to reduce inflammation in the body. Chronic inflammation has been linked to a number of chronic diseases, including heart disease, diabetes, and cancer.

5. Environmental sustainability: A plant-based diet is more sustainable for the environment, as it requires fewer resources to produce plant-based foods compared to animal-based foods. Animal agriculture is a major contributor to greenhouse gas emissions, deforestation, and water pollution.

6. Ethical considerations: For many people, following a plant-based diet is also an ethical choice, as it avoids the exploitation and suffering of animals for food production.

Overall, a plant-based diet can provide numerous health benefits while also being more sustainable and ethical. It is important to ensure that you are getting all of the necessary nutrients from your diet, however, so it may be helpful to consult with a registered dietitian to ensure that you are meeting your nutritional needs.

Key Ingredients and Seasonings

A plant-based diet is based on whole, minimally processed foods derived from plants. Here are some key ingredients and seasonings that are commonly used in plant-based cooking:

1. Fruits and vegetables: These are the foundation of a plant-based diet. They provide a wide range of vitamins, minerals, and antioxidants, as well as fiber for healthy digestion. Some popular fruits and vegetables include leafy greens, berries, citrus fruits, tomatoes, peppers, carrots, and sweet potatoes.

2. Whole grains: Whole grains are an important source of complex carbohydrates, which provide energy and help to keep you feeling full. They also contain fiber, vitamins, and minerals.

Some examples of whole grains include brown rice, quinoa, oats, and whole wheat bread.

3. Legumes: Legumes, such as beans, lentils, and chickpeas, are a great source of plant-based protein. They are also high in fiber, iron, and other nutrients. Legumes can be used in a variety of dishes, including soups, stews, salads, and dips.

4. Nuts and seeds: Nuts and seeds are a good source of healthy fats, protein, and fiber. They can be eaten as a snack or used as a topping for salads, oatmeal, or yogurt. Some popular nuts and seeds include almonds, walnuts, chia seeds, and flaxseeds.

5. Herbs and spices: Herbs and spices can add flavor and depth to plant-based dishes without adding extra calories or salt. Some popular herbs and spices include basil, oregano, rosemary, cumin, and turmeric.

6. Plant-based milks: Plant-based milks, such as almond milk, soy milk, and coconut milk, can be used in place of dairy milk in recipes. They are lower in calories and saturated fat than dairy milk, and are a good source of calcium and vitamin D.

Overall, a plant-based diet is based on a wide variety of whole, minimally processed foods derived from plants. By incorporating these key ingredients and seasonings into your cooking, you can create flavorful and nutritious meals that support your health and well-being.

Tips for Maintaining a Healthy Eating Habit

Maintaining a plant-based diet can be challenging at first, but with some planning and preparation, it can become a sustainable and enjoyable way of eating. Here are some tips for maintaining a plant-based diet:

1. Plan your meals: Take some time each week to plan out your meals and snacks. This will help you stay on track and avoid reaching for unhealthy convenience foods.

2. Stock up on plant-based staples: Keep your pantry and fridge stocked with plant-based staples such as whole grains, legumes, fruits, vegetables, nuts, and seeds. This will make it easier to whip up healthy meals and snacks.

3. Experiment with new recipes: Try out new plant-based recipes to keep things interesting and prevent boredom. There are many plant-based recipe websites and cookbooks available for inspiration.

4. Focus on nutrient-dense foods: Make sure that you are getting all of the necessary nutrients from your diet by focusing on nutrient-dense foods such as leafy greens, berries, whole grains, and legumes.

5. Be mindful of protein intake: While plant-based diets can provide plenty of protein, it is important to be mindful of your intake and make sure that you are getting enough. Good sources of plant-based protein include beans, lentils, tofu, tempeh, nuts, and seeds.

6. Don't forget about healthy fats: Healthy fats are an important part of a balanced diet and can be found in foods such as avocados, nuts, seeds, and olive oil.

7. Stay hydrated: Drinking plenty of water is important for overall health and can also help to keep you feeling full and satisfied.

8. Don't be too hard on yourself: Remember that it's okay to slip up or have an occasional indulgence. The key is to focus on progress, not perfection, and to make sustainable changes over time.

Cooking Techniques

Cooking plant-based meals can be a fun and creative experience. Here are some cooking techniques that can help you make delicious and nutritious plant-based dishes:

1. Roasting: Roasting is a great way to bring out the natural sweetness of vegetables. Simply toss your veggies with some olive oil, salt, and pepper, and roast them in the oven until they are tender and caramelized.

2. Steaming: Steaming is a gentle cooking method that helps to preserve the nutrients in your food. This technique works well for vegetables such as broccoli, cauliflower, and carrots.

3. Sautéing: Sautéing involves cooking food quickly over high heat in a small amount of oil or water. This technique works well for vegetables, tofu, and tempeh.

4. Stir-frying: Stir-frying involves cooking food quickly over high heat in a wok or skillet. This technique works well for vegetables, tofu, and tempeh, and can be seasoned with soy sauce, ginger, garlic, and other flavorful ingredients.

5. Grilling: Grilling is a great way to add smoky flavor to vegetables, tofu, and tempeh. Simply brush your food with a little oil and seasonings, and grill until charred and tender.

6. Baking: Baking is a versatile cooking method that can be used for everything from casseroles to desserts. Plant-based baked goods can be made with ingredients such as almond flour, coconut oil, and flax eggs.

7. Blending: Blending is a great way to make smoothies, soups, and sauces. A high-speed blender can easily blend fruits, vegetables, and nuts into creamy and delicious concoctions.

Overall, there are many different cooking techniques that can be used to create delicious and nutritious plant-based meals. Experiment with different methods and ingredients to find what works best for you.

Essential Kitchen Tools

Cooking plant-based meals can be simple and enjoyable with the right kitchen tools. Here are some essential kitchen tools for cooking a plant-based diet:

1. High-speed blender: A high-speed blender is great for making smoothies, soups, sauces, and nut butters.

2. Food processor: A food processor is useful for chopping vegetables, making dips and spreads, and grinding nuts and seeds.

3. Vegetable peeler: A vegetable peeler is essential for peeling vegetables and fruits quickly and easily.

4. Chef's knife: A sharp chef's knife is important for chopping vegetables and fruits with ease.

5. Cutting board: A sturdy cutting board is necessary for chopping vegetables, fruits, and herbs.

6. Non-stick skillet: A non-stick skillet is great for sautéing vegetables without using too much oil.

7. Baking sheets: Baking sheets are useful for roasting vegetables and baking plant-based goods such as cookies and granola.

8. Steamer basket: A steamer basket is great for steaming vegetables, tofu, and tempeh.

9. Colander: A colander is necessary for draining and rinsing grains, legumes, and vegetables.

10. Mason jars: Mason jars are great for storing leftovers, homemade dressings, and smoothies.

By having these essential kitchen tools on hand, you can easily prepare healthy and delicious plant-based meals at home.

Meal Planning and Prepping

Meal planning and preparation are important components of maintaining a healthy plant-based diet. Here are some tips to help you plan and prepare your meals:

1. Plan your meals ahead of time: Take some time each week to plan out your meals and snacks. This will help you stay on track and avoid reaching for unhealthy convenience foods.

2. Make a grocery list: Once you have planned your meals, make a grocery list to ensure that you have all of the necessary ingredients on hand.

3. Prep your ingredients in advance: Spend some time prepping your ingredients in advance, such as washing and chopping vegetables or cooking grains and legumes. This can save you time during the week and make it easier to whip up healthy meals.

4. Batch cook: Consider batch cooking large batches of grains, legumes, or soups at the beginning of the week, so that you have meals ready to go throughout the week.

5. Use meal prep containers: Invest in some meal prep containers to portion out your meals and snacks in advance. This can help you stay on track with your eating goals and prevent overeating.

6. Keep healthy snacks on hand: Stock your pantry and fridge with healthy plant-based snacks such as fresh fruit, raw veggies, hummus, and nuts.

7. Experiment with new recipes: Try out new plant-based recipes to keep things interesting and prevent boredom. There are many plant-based recipe websites and cookbooks available for inspiration.

8. Don't forget about convenience foods: While it's best to focus on whole, minimally processed foods, there are also many healthy convenience foods available, such as frozen vegetables, canned beans, and pre-packaged salads.

By taking the time to plan and prepare your meals in advance, you can make it easier to stick to a healthy plant-based diet and enjoy delicious and nutritious meals throughout the week.

Tips for Dining out and Travelling on a plant-based Diet

Maintaining a plant-based diet while dining out or traveling can be challenging, but it is definitely possible. Here are some tips to help you navigate these situations:

Dining Out:

1. Research restaurants in advance: Look up menus online before going out to eat to see if there are any plant-based options available.

2. Ask for modifications: Don't be afraid to ask your server to modify dishes to make them plant-based. For example, you can ask for no cheese on a salad or for tofu instead of meat in a stir-fry.

3. Choose ethnic cuisines: Many ethnic cuisines, such as Indian, Thai, and Ethiopian, have a variety of plant-based options.

4. Order side dishes: If there are no plant-based entrees on the menu, consider ordering a few side dishes to create a meal.

5. Be prepared with snacks: Bring along healthy plant-based snacks, such as nuts, seeds, and fruit, in case there are no suitable options available.

Traveling:

1. Pack healthy snacks: Bring along healthy plant-based snacks, such as energy bars, dried fruit, and nuts, to keep you fueled throughout the day.

2. Research restaurants in advance: Look up plant-based restaurants or vegan-friendly options in the area you will be visiting.

3. Consider renting an apartment: If you have access to a kitchen, you can prepare your own plant-based meals using local ingredients.

4. Visit local markets: Explore local markets to find fresh fruits, vegetables, and other plant-based ingredients.

5. Be flexible: While it's important to stick to your plant-based diet as much as possible, it's also important to be flexible and enjoy new experiences. Don't stress too much if you can't find plant-based options at every meal.

By being prepared and doing some research in advance, you can maintain a healthy plant-based diet while dining out or traveling.

30-Day Meal Plan

DAYS	BREAKFAST	LUNCH	DINNER	SNACK/DESSERT
1	Pan con Tomate P 11	Lucky Black-Eyed Pea Stew P 28	Sheet-Pan Garlicky Kale P 48	Vanilla Bean Whip P 37
2	Potato and Veggie Breakfast Casserole ✗ P 11	Chickpea Pâté P 28	Steamed Kabocha Squash with Nori and Scallions P 53	Almond Anise Biscotti P 37
3	Mango Ginger Kombucha Mimosas P 11	Tahini Green Beans P 29	Baby Potatoes with Dill, Chives, and Garlic P 52	Almond-Date Energy Bites P 37
4	Sunshine Muffins P 14	Nut-Crusted Tofu P 29	Blackened Sprouts P 52	Banana Soft Serve P 38
5	Blueberry and Peanut Butter Parfait Bowls P 14	Quinoa Primavera P 28	Vegetable Spring Rolls with Spicy Peanut Dipping Sauce P 49	Caramel-Coconut Frosted Brownies P 38
6	Overnight Pumpkin Spice Chia Pudding P 12	Mango Satay Tempeh Bowl P 29	Jicama-Citrus Pickle P 53	Zesty Orange-Cranberry Energy Bites P 38
7	Cherry Pecan Granola Bars P 12	Orzo "Risotto" P 30	Lemony Steamed Kale with Olives P 52	Pumpkin Spice Bread P 39
8	Tempeh Breakfast Sausage P 12	Chickpea Tortilla Fajita Stack P 30	Cumin-Citrus Roasted Carrots P 51	Blueberry-Lime Sorbet P 39
9	Almond and Protein Shake P 13	Baked Tempeh Nuggets P 31	Avocado Tartare P 50	No-Bake Mocha Cheesecake P 41
10	Savory Quinoa Breakfast Cups P 13	Red Lentil Pâté P 28	Ratatouille P 48	Nice Cream P 40
11	Roasted Root Vegetable Hash P 13	Garlic Mashed Potatoes P 46	Green Mix Salad P 68	Cherry Chocolate Bark P 39
12	Banana, Date and Coconut Muesli P 14	Zucchini "Parmesan" P 46	Tomato, Corn and Bean Salad P 69	Apple Crisp P 42
13	Sweet Potato Toasts with Avocado Mash and Tahini P 13	Teriyaki Mushrooms P 47	Lentil, Lemon and Mushroom Salad P 70	Mango Sticky Rice P 41
14	Fruit Salad with Zesty Citrus Couscous P 15	Yellow Bell Pepper Boats P 46	Apple Broccoli Crunch Bowl P 70	Two-Minute Turtles P 41
15	Best Whole Wheat Pancakes P 15	Savory Sweet Potato Casserole P 46	Greek Salad in a Jar P 71	Pumpkin Bread Pudding P 38
16	Maple-Spice Buckwheat Crispies Cereal P 14	Vegan Goulash P 48	Forbidden Black Rice and Edamame Salad P 72	Protein Peanut Butter Balls P 56

DAYS	BREAKFAST	LUNCH	DINNER	SNACK/DESSERT
17	Grain-Free Porridge P 15	Fennel and Cherry Tomato Gratin P 48	Mock Tuna Salad P 67	Slow Cooker Chipotle Tacos P 56
18	Spring Breakfast Salad P 18	Broccolini on Fire P 53	Fiery Couscous Salad P 73	Savory Roasted Chickpeas P 56
19	Maca-Mint Smoothie P 11	Spicy Butternut Squash Bisque P 47	Bulgur Lettuce Cups P 75	Orange Cranberry Power Cookies P 56
20	Cleansing Morning Lemonade P 18	Stir-Fried Vegetables with Miso and Sake P 47	Vegan "Toona" Salad P 71	Mango Plantain Nice Cream P 57
21	Ful Medames (Egyptian Breakfast Beans) P 17	Cabbage Salad and Peanut Butter Vinaigrette P 67	North African Chickpeas and Vegetables P 32	Oat Crunch Apple Crisp P 57
22	Paradise Island Overnight Oatmeal P 18	Tuscan White Bean Salad P 67	Chana Saag P 32	Sunshine Everything Crackers P 57
23	Breakfast Hummus on Toast P 16	Kale, Black Bean and Quinoa Salad P 67	Mixed Beans Chili P 32	Sesame-Tamari Portable Rice Balls P 58
24	Maple, Apple, and Walnut Great Grains P 11	Succotash Salad P 68	Farro Tabbouleh P 34	Loaded Sweet Apple "Nachos" P 58
25	Vanilla Protein Pancakes P 16	Mango Lentil Salad P 68	Hearty Veggie Hoagies P 34	Baked Vegetable Chips P 59
26	Spelt Berry Hot Breakfast Cereal P 59	Quinoa Arugula Salad P 68	Mexican Quinoa Bowl P 34	Peanut Butter Snack Squares P 58
27	Warm Maple Protein Oatmeal P 12	Fava Bean Salad P 69	Bulgur Chickpea Pilaf P 33	Pump Up the Power Energy Balls P 59
28	Overnight Muesli P 16	Warm Lentil Salad P 69	Fancy Rice P 33	Tortilla Chips P 61
29	Red Flannel Beet Hash with Dill P 17	Strawberry-Pistachio Salad P 69	Lentil-Mushroom No-Meat Pasta (Bolognese) P 30	White Bean Caponata P 59
30	Apple Cinnamon Oats Bowl P 18	Warm Sweet Potato and Brussels Sprout Salad P 68	Mujadara (Lentils with Rice and Caramelized Onions) P 33	Toast Points P 60

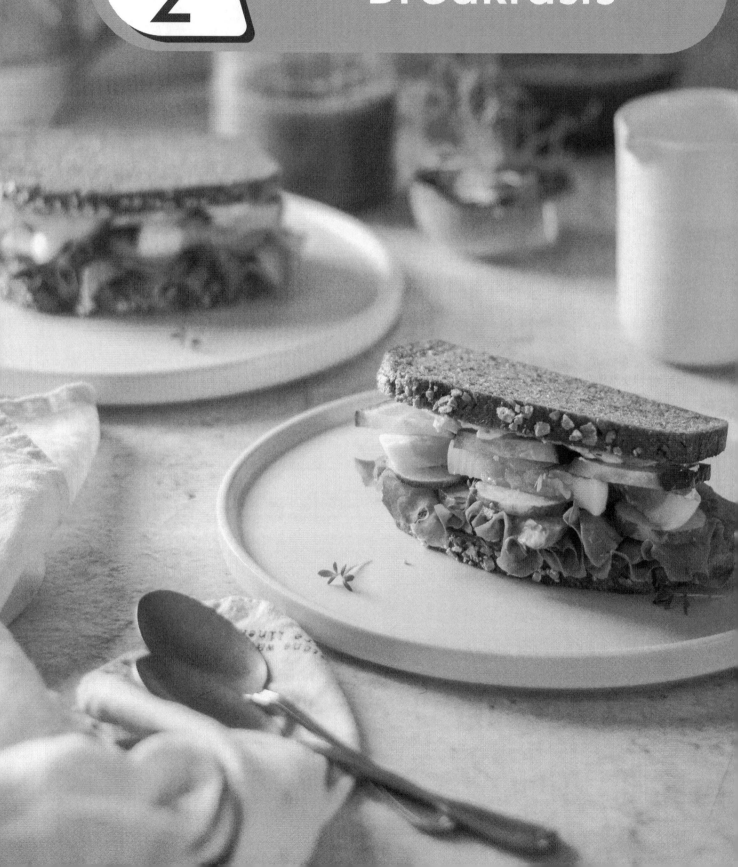

Chapter 2
Breakfasts

Pan con Tomate

Prep time: 5 minutes | Cook time: 0 minutes | Makes 2 slices

2 large slices toast
1 garlic clove, halved
1 Roma tomato, halved
Salt (optional)
Nutritional yeast (optional)

1. Take each slice of toast and rub it with a half of a garlic clove and half of a Roma tomato. Then, sprinkle with salt and, if you prefer, nutritional yeast.

Per Serving: (1 slice)
calories: 90 | fat: 1g | protein: 3g | carbs: 17g | fiber: 2g

Maca-Mint Smoothie

Prep time: 2 minutes | Cook time: 0 minutes | Serves 1

2 tablespoons raw cashews
1 heaping handful of baby spinach
1 cup almond mylk
2 frozen bananas, chopped
1 tablespoon fresh lemon juice
20 fresh mint leaves
1 teaspoon maca powder
1 tablespoon cacao nibs (optional)

1. Place all the ingredients, except for the cacao nibs, into a high-speed blender.
2. Blend the ingredients until they are smooth and creamy.
3. If desired, sprinkle the cacao nibs on top as a topping.

Per Serving:
calories: 554 | fat: 37g | protein: 10g | carbs: 55g | fiber: 10g

Potato and Veggie Breakfast Casserole 8/3

Prep time: 10 minutes | Cook time: 4 to 5 hours | Serves 4 to 6

1 medium red bell pepper, diced
1 medium onion, diced
1 (8-ounce / 227-g) package white button or cremini mushrooms, quartered
3 cups chopped kale
Ground black pepper
Salt (optional)
1 teaspoon garlic powder, divided
1 teaspoon onion powder, divided
1 teaspoon paprika, divided
1 (14-ounce / 397-g) package extra-firm tofu, drained
1 teaspoon ground turmeric
8 small Yukon Gold or red potatoes (about 2 pounds / 907 g), unpeeled and sliced into half-inch rounds

1. In the slow cooker, place the bell pepper, onion, mushrooms, and kale. Season with pepper and, if desired, salt. Add ½ teaspoon each of garlic powder, onion powder, and paprika. Mix well to distribute the seasonings. 2. Crumble the tofu directly into the slow cooker, and sprinkle with turmeric. Stir until the tofu is coated and combined with the veggies. 3. Layer the potatoes on top of the tofu and veggies. Sprinkle with the remaining ½ teaspoon each of garlic powder, onion powder, and paprika. Season with salt and pepper again, if desired. Cover and cook on High for 4 to 5 hours or on Low for 7 to 8 hours.

Per Serving:
calories: 334 | fat: 6g | protein: 18g | carbs: 54g | fiber: 7g

Mango Ginger Kombucha Mimosas

Prep time: 10 minutes | Cook time: 5 minutes | Serves 8

1 cup chopped fresh mango or thawed frozen mango chunks
1 piece of fresh ginger, peeled and minced
2 tablespoons filtered water
½ teaspoon pure maple syrup (optional)
1 tablespoon fresh lime juice
3 cups ginger-flavored kombucha, chilled
8 lime wedges, for serving

1. In a medium saucepan over medium heat, combine the mango, ginger, water, and maple syrup, if using. Bring it to a boil and then reduce the heat to a simmer. Cook until the mango becomes soft and mushy, which usually takes about 3 minutes. Transfer the contents of the saucepan into a blender. 2. Add the lime juice to the blender and blend on high speed until you obtain a smooth purée. If desired, you can strain the purée to remove any solids. 3. Pour 1 tablespoon of mango purée into each glass. Divide the ginger kombucha evenly among the glasses. Serve each drink with a lime wedge.

Per Serving:
calories: 32 | fat: 0g | protein: 1g | carbs: 3g | fiber: 0g

Maple, Apple, and Walnut Great Grains

Prep time: 10 minutes | Cook time: 3 to 4 hours | Serves 4 to 6

2 large apples
½ cup quinoa, rinsed
½ cup steel-cut oats
½ cup wheat berries
½ cup pearl barley
½ cup bulgur wheat
1 tablespoon ground flaxseed
2 teaspoons ground cinnamon
½ teaspoon ground or grated nutmeg
7 cups water
⅓ cup maple syrup (optional)
½ cup chopped walnuts
½ cup raisins
Unsweetened plant-based milk, for serving (optional)

1. Peel, core, and chop the apples and place them in the slow cooker. Add the quinoa, oats, wheat berries, barley, bulgur wheat, flaxseed, cinnamon, nutmeg, water, and maple syrup (if using). Stir gently. Cover and cook on High for 3 to 4 hours or on Low for 7 to 8 hours. 2. Before serving, stir in the walnuts and raisins. Spoon into a bowl and add your favorite milk (if using).

Per Serving:
calories: 691 | fat: 13g | protein: 18g | carbs: 113g | fiber: 21g

Powerhouse Protein Shake

Prep time: 5 minutes | Cook time: 0 minutes | Serves 2

2 green apples, peeled, cored, and chopped
1 cup fresh or frozen pineapple chunks
1 cup fresh kale, chopped
1 cup spinach, drained and rinsed
1 teaspoon spirulina
1 cup coconut water
2 scoops of unflavored vegan protein powder

1. Add all the required ingredients to a blender. Blend for 2 minutes. Transfer to a large cup or shaker. Enjoy!

Per Serving:
calories: 257 | fat: 4g | protein: 26g | carbs: 30g | fiber: 5g

Overnight Pumpkin Spice Chia Pudding

Prep time: 10 minutes | Cook time: 0 minutes | Serves 4

¾ cup chia seeds
2 cups unsweetened plant-based milk
1 (15-ounce / 425-g) can unsweetened pumpkin purée
¼ cup maple syrup (optional)
1 tablespoon pumpkin pie spice blend
1 cup water
½ cup pecans, for serving

1. Whisk together chia seeds, plant-based milk, pumpkin purée, maple syrup (if desired), pumpkin pie spice, and water in a large bowl. 2. Divide the mixture evenly among 4 mason jars or containers with lids. Allow it to sit for 10 minutes, then stir each container to ensure there are no clumps of chia. Cover the jars and refrigerate overnight to allow the mixture to firm up. When ready to serve, garnish each jar with a sprinkle of pecans.

Per Serving:
calories: 421 | fat: 23g | protein: 12g | carbs: 47g | fiber: 20g

Cherry Pecan Granola Bars

Prep time: 10 minutes | Cook time: 45 minutes | Makes 12 bars

2 cups rolled oats
½ cup dates, pitted and coarsely chopped
½ cup orange juice
¼ cup chopped pecans
1 cup fruit-sweetened dried cherries
½ teaspoon ground cinnamon
¼ teaspoon ground allspice
Pinch salt, or to taste (optional)

1. Preheat the oven to 325ºF (165ºC). 2. Spread the oats evenly on a baking sheet measuring 13 × 18 inches and bake for approximately 10 minutes, or until they turn slightly golden. Remove from the oven and transfer the toasted oats to a large mixing bowl. 3. In a small saucepan, combine the dates and orange juice. Cook over medium-low heat for about 15 minutes, until the dates soften. Transfer the mixture to a blender and process until it becomes smooth and creamy. 4. Add the date mixture to the bowl with the oats. Also add the pecans, dried cherries, cinnamon, allspice, and salt (if desired). Mix everything together until well combined. 5. Press the mixture firmly into a nonstick baking pan measuring 8 × 8 inches. Bake for approximately 20 minutes, or until the top turns lightly golden. Allow the bars to cool before slicing them into desired portions.

Per Serving:
calories: 92 | fat: 2g | protein: 3g | carbs: 20g | fiber: 3g

Tempeh Breakfast Sausage

Prep time: 15 minutes | Cook time: 20 minutes | Makes 12 patties

1 (8-ounce / 227-g) package tempeh, lightly steamed and cubed
2 tablespoons maple syrup (optional)
2 tablespoons whole wheat flour
2 tablespoons vegetable broth
1 tablespoon red miso
1 teaspoon dried sage
½ teaspoon dried rosemary
¼ teaspoon black pepper
⅛ teaspoon crushed red pepper

1. Preheat the oven to 400ºF (205ºC) and line a baking sheet with parchment paper.
2. In the bowl of a food processor, combine the tempeh, maple syrup (if desired), flour, broth, miso, sage, rosemary, black pepper, and crushed red pepper. Pulse the ingredients until well combined. 3. Transfer the mixture to a medium-sized bowl. Using wet hands, shape the mixture into 12 slider-sized patties. 4. Place the patties onto the prepared baking sheet and bake for 20 minutes, flipping them halfway through cooking. Once done, serve the sausage patties. (The leftovers can be refrigerated for up to 5 days.)

Per Serving: (1 patty)
calories: 53 | fat: 2g | protein: 4g | carbs: 5g | fiber: 0g

Warm Maple Protein Oatmeal

Prep time: 5 minutes | Cook time: 30 minutes | Serves 2

1 cup steel-cut oats
3 tablespoons raw shelled hempseed, divided
3 tablespoons maple syrup (optional)
2 teaspoons cinnamon
1 tablespoon slivered almonds
1 tablespoon currants

1. Bring 4 cups of water to a boil in a large saucepan. Add the steel-cut oatmeal, 2 tablespoons hempseed, maple syrup (if desired), and cinnamon and bring back to a boil. Reduce heat to low and cook uncovered for 30 minutes, stirring occasionally. 2. Serve in bowls, garnished with almond slivers, currants, and the remaining hempseed.

Per Serving:
calories: 229 | fat: 6g | protein: 23g | carbs: 47g | fiber: 9g

Savory Quinoa Breakfast Cups

Prep time: 10 minutes | Cook time: 40 minutes | Serves 6

½ cup plus 3 tablespoons quinoa
½ cup spinach
½ cup sliced mushrooms
1 cup diary-free milk
⅓ cup chickpea flour
1 tablespoon nutritional yeast
2 tablespoons raw shelled hempseed
½ teaspoon salt (optional)

1. Begin by rinsing the quinoa thoroughly using a sieve. In a small saucepan, combine the quinoa with 1 cup plus 2 tablespoons of water. Bring it to a boil, then cover and reduce the heat to a simmer. Let it cook for about 10 to 15 minutes or until all the liquid is absorbed. Remove from heat and let it sit, covered, for an additional 5 minutes. Remove the lid and fluff the quinoa with a fork. 2. Preheat the oven to 375ºF (190ºC). 3. Line a six-cup muffin tin with paper muffin cups. 4. Place the spinach and mushrooms in a food processor and process until finely chopped. 5. In a large bowl, combine all the ingredients, including the processed spinach and mushrooms. Mix well to ensure everything is evenly incorporated. 6. Divide the mixture equally among the muffin cups. Bake for approximately 20 to 25 minutes.

Per Serving:
calories: 123 | fat: 3g | protein: 7g | carbs: 17g | fiber: 2g

Roasted Root Vegetable Hash

Prep time: 15 minutes | Cook time: 30 minutes | Serves 4

2 teaspoons extra-virgin olive oil (optional)
1 small yellow onion, cut into ½-inch pieces
½ medium butternut squash, peeled, seeded, and cut into 1½-inch cubes
2 large carrots, peeled and cut into 1-inch rounds
2 medium sweet potatoes, cut into 1½-inch cubes
2 medium yellow potatoes, cut into 1½-inch cubes
1 bunch small red or pink radishes, trimmed and halved
1 teaspoon garlic powder
1 teaspoon smoked paprika
1 teaspoon salt (optional)
4 tablespoons plain plant-based yogurt, for serving
1 avocado, peeled, pitted, quartered, and thinly sliced, for serving
Black pepper

1. Preheat the oven to 400ºF (205ºC). Grease a sheet pan with olive oil, ensuring it is evenly spread across the surface. 2. In a bowl, combine the onion, butternut squash, carrots, sweet potatoes, yellow potatoes, and radishes. Sprinkle garlic powder, smoked paprika, and salt over the vegetables. Toss the vegetables with your hands until they are coated evenly with the oil and spices. 3. Spread the vegetable mixture on the greased sheet pan. Bake for 20 minutes. Then, using a spatula, flip the vegetables and bake for an additional 10 minutes, or until they can be easily pierced with a fork. 4. Divide the hash among plates and top each portion with 1 tablespoon of yogurt, a quarter of the avocado slices, and black pepper to taste.

Per Serving:
calories: 325 | fat: 10g | protein: 7g | carbs: 56g | fiber: 12g

Sweet Potato Toasts with Avocado Mash and Tahini

Prep time: 10 minutes | Cook time: 30 minutes | Serves 4

Sweet Potato Toasts:
Olive oil cooking spray
4 medium sweet potatoes
Pinch of salt (optional)
Avocado Mash:
2 medium avocados, pitted and peeled
Juice of ½ lemon
Pinch of salt (optional)
Serve:
2 ounces (57 g) arugula (about 2 cups)
8 teaspoons tahini
8 teaspoons hemp hearts
Pinch red pepper flakes (optional)

1. To make the Sweet Potato Toasts, preheat the oven to 400ºF (205ºC) and lightly coat a sheet pan with olive oil cooking spray. 2. Slice the sweet potatoes lengthwise into ½-inch-thick slices, resulting in approximately 4 slices per potato. 3. Arrange the sweet potato slices in a single layer on the prepared sheet pan and sprinkle them with salt. Bake for 15 minutes, then flip the slices over and continue baking for another 15 minutes, or until the potatoes are slightly browned, crispy on the outside, and soft in the middle. 4. For the Avocado Mash, use a fork to mash the avocados in a bowl. Add lemon juice and salt (if desired), and stir until well combined. 5. To assemble the toasts, spread about 1 teaspoon of avocado mash onto each sweet potato slice. Top each toast with approximately 5 arugula leaves, drizzle with ½ teaspoon of tahini, and sprinkle with ½ teaspoon of hemp hearts. If desired, add a pinch of red pepper flakes for some extra spice.

Per Serving:
calories: 375 | fat: 23g | protein: 7g | carbs: 38g | fiber: 12g

Almond and Protein Shake

Prep time: 5 minutes | Cook time: 0 minutes | Serves 2

1½ cups soy milk
3 tablespoons almonds
1 teaspoon maple syrup (optional)
1 tablespoon coconut oil (optional)
2 scoops of chocolate or vanilla flavor vegan protein powder
2 to 4 ice cubes
1 teaspoon cocoa powder (optional)

1. Place all the necessary ingredients, along with the optional cocoa powder if desired, into a blender. Blend for approximately 2 minutes until well combined and smooth. 2. Pour the shake into a large cup or shaker. Serve and enjoy!

Per Serving:
calories: 340 | fat: 17g | protein: 32g | carbs: 15g | fiber: 2g

Sunshine Muffins

Prep time: 15 minutes | Cook time: 30 minutes | Makes 6 muffins

1 teaspoon coconut oil, for greasing muffin tins (optional)
2 tablespoons almond butter or sunflower seed butter
¼ cup nondairy milk
1 orange, peeled
1 carrot, coarsely chopped
2 tablespoons chopped dried apricots or other dried fruit
3 tablespoons molasses
2 tablespoons ground flaxseed
1 teaspoon apple cider vinegar
1 teaspoon pure vanilla extract
½ teaspoon ground cinnamon
½ teaspoon ground ginger (optional)
¼ teaspoon ground nutmeg (optional)
¼ teaspoon allspice (optional)
¾ cup rolled oats or whole-grain flour
1 teaspoon baking powder
½ teaspoon baking soda
Mix-Ins (optional):
½ cup rolled oats
2 tablespoons raisins or other chopped dried fruit
2 tablespoons sunflower seeds

1. Preheat the oven to 350ºF (180ºC). Prepare a 6-cup muffin tin by greasing the cups with coconut oil (if desired) or using silicone or paper muffin cups. 2. In a food processor or blender, blend together the nut butter, milk, orange, carrot, apricots, molasses, flaxseed, vinegar, vanilla, cinnamon, ginger, nutmeg, and allspice until they form a somewhat smooth purée. 3. Grind the oats in a clean coffee grinder until they reach a flour-like consistency (or use whole-grain flour). In a large bowl, combine the ground oats with the baking powder and baking soda. 4. Gently mix the wet ingredients into the dry ingredients until just combined. If desired, fold in any additional mix-ins. 5. Spoon approximately ¼ cup of batter into each muffin cup and bake for about 30 minutes, or until a toothpick inserted into the center comes out clean. Note that the presence of orange in the batter may make the muffins more moist, so depending on the weight of your muffin tin, they may require additional baking time.

Per Serving: (1 muffin)
calories: 226 | fat: 8g | protein: 7g | carbs: 34g | fiber: 6g

Blueberry and Peanut Butter Parfait Bowls

Prep time: 10 minutes | Cook time: 0 minutes | Serves 2

2 cups plain plant-based yogurt
1 cup store-bought granola
2 tablespoons maple syrup (optional)
½ cup fresh blueberries
2 tablespoons roughly chopped walnuts
2 tablespoons natural peanut butter

1. Take 2 bowls and evenly distribute the yogurt between them. Sprinkle half of the granola on top of each bowl and if desired, drizzle with 1 tablespoon of maple syrup. 2. Add half of the blueberries, 1 tablespoon of walnuts, and 1 tablespoon of peanut butter to each bowl as toppings.

Per Serving:
calories: 567 | fat: 24g | protein: 17g | carbs: 75g | fiber: 13g

Banana, Date and Coconut Muesli

Prep time: 10 minutes | Cook time: 0 minutes | Serves 2

1 cup rolled oats
¾ cup unsweetened almond milk
½ cup pitted and chopped dates
¼ cup unsweetened coconut, toasted
1 banana, peeled and sliced

1. In a bowl mix all ingredients and let soak 15 minutes.

Per Serving:
calories: 331 | fat: 7g | protein: 13g | carbs: 76g | fiber: 12g

Maple-Spice Buckwheat Crispies Cereal

Prep time: 15 minutes | Cook time: 50 minutes | Makes 5 cups

1 cup raw buckwheat groats, soaked for at least 1 hour
1 cup sliced almonds
1 cup large-flake coconut
½ cup raw sunflower seeds
2 tablespoons chia seeds
3 tablespoons maple sugar or coconut sugar (optional)
¼ teaspoon fine sea salt (optional)
1½ teaspoons ground cinnamon
¼ teaspoon ground ginger
¼ teaspoon ground nutmeg
2 tablespoons liquid virgin coconut oil
¼ cup pure maple syrup (optional)
1 teaspoon pure vanilla extract

1. Preheat the oven to 325ºF (165ºC) and line a large baking sheet with parchment paper. 2. Place a clean kitchen towel or doubled paper towels on a flat surface. Rinse the buckwheat groats thoroughly in a fine-mesh strainer, removing as much of the slimy soaking liquid as possible. Spread the rinsed buckwheat groats onto the towel and pat them dry lightly. Transfer the dried buckwheat groats to a large bowl. 3. Add sliced almonds, coconut flakes, sunflower seeds, chia seeds, maple sugar, sea salt (if desired), cinnamon, ginger, and nutmeg to the bowl with the buckwheat groats. Toss everything together to coat evenly. 4. In a small bowl, whisk together coconut oil, maple syrup (if desired), and vanilla extract. Pour the mixture over the buckwheat groats mixture and stir with a rubber spatula until well coated. 5. Scrape the wet cereal mixture onto the prepared baking sheet. Use the back of the spatula to flatten and spread it out as much as possible. Place the baking sheet in the oven and bake for 50 minutes, stirring and flipping the crispies a few times during cooking to ensure even browning. Once the cereal is evenly golden brown and lightly crispy, it is ready. 6. Allow the cereal to cool completely before storing it in a sealed container at room temperature. This cereal will stay fresh for about 10 days.

Per Serving: (½ cup)
calories: 195 | fat: 14g | protein: 4g | carbs: 16g | fiber: 3g

Fruit Salad with Zesty Citrus Couscous

Prep time: 5 minutes | Cook time: 5 minutes | Serves 1

1 orange, zested and juiced
¼ cup whole wheat couscous or corn couscous
1 cup assorted berries (strawberries, blackberries, blueberries)
½ cup cubed or balled melon (cantaloupe or honeydew)
1 tablespoon maple syrup or coconut sugar (optional)
1 tablespoon fresh mint, minced (optional)
1 tablespoon unsweetened coconut flakes

1. In a small pot, bring the orange juice and half of the zest to a boil. 2. Place the dry couscous in a small bowl and pour the boiling orange juice over it. If the juice is not enough to fully submerge the couscous, add just enough boiling water to cover it. Cover the bowl with a plate or wrap it tightly, and let it steep for 5 minutes. 3. In a medium bowl, combine the berries and melon. Toss them with maple syrup (if desired) and the remaining zest. You can either keep the fruit cool or lightly heat it in the same small pot used for the orange juice. 4. Once the couscous has softened, remove the cover and fluff it with a fork. Top the couscous with the prepared fruit mixture, fresh mint, and coconut.

Per Serving:
calories: 258 | fat: 2g | protein: 4g | carbs: 59g | fiber: 7g

Best Whole Wheat Pancakes

Prep time: 10 minutes | Cook time: 20 minutes | Serves 4

3 tablespoons ground flaxseed
6 tablespoons warm water
1½ cups whole wheat pastry flour
½ cup rye flour
2 tablespoons double-acting baking powder
1 teaspoon ground cinnamon
½ teaspoon ground ginger
1½ cups unsweetened nondairy milk
3 tablespoons pure maple syrup (optional)
1 teaspoon vanilla extract

1. In a small bowl, mix together the flaxseed and warm water. Set it aside for at least 5 minutes to thicken. 2. In a large bowl, whisk together the pastry flour, rye flour, baking powder, cinnamon, and ginger until well combined. 3. In a glass measuring cup, whisk together the milk, maple syrup (if desired), and vanilla extract. Using a spatula, gently fold the wet ingredients into the dry ingredients. Add the soaked flaxseed mixture and continue folding until everything is fully incorporated. 4. Heat a large skillet or nonstick griddle over medium-high heat. Working in batches of 3 to 4 pancakes at a time, pour ¼-cup portions of batter onto the hot skillet. Cook for approximately 3 to 4 minutes per side, or until the pancakes are golden brown and there is no visible liquid batter left.

Per Serving: (3 pancakes)
calories: 301 | fat: 4g | protein: 10g | carbs: 57g | fiber: 10g

Grain-Free Porridge

Prep time: 10 minutes | Cook time: 20 minutes | Makes 3½ cups

½ cup whole raw almonds, soaked overnight in 2 cups filtered water
3 cups filtered water
¼ cup coconut flour
Pinch of fine sea salt (optional)
½ cup raw sunflower seeds, soaked overnight in 2 cups filtered water
½ cup unsweetened flaked dried coconut
3 tablespoons whole flaxseeds
2 tablespoons chia seeds

1. Start by draining and rinsing the almonds. Transfer them to an upright blender. Add 3 cups of water, coconut flour, and salt (if desired). Blend until you achieve a smooth consistency. 2. Drain and rinse the sunflower seeds, then add them to the blender along with the coconut. Pulse until the seeds and coconut are coarsely ground. 3. Pour the mixture into a medium-sized pot and bring it to a boil over high heat, whisking frequently. 4. Remove the pot from the heat and whisk in the flax and chia seeds until thoroughly combined. Cover the porridge and set it aside for 5 minutes to allow it to thicken. 5. Give the porridge a final whisk before serving. If there are any leftovers, pour them into a wide-mouthed glass jar or another container. Allow the porridge to cool, then cover tightly and store it in the refrigerator for up to 4 days.

Per Serving: (½ cup)
calories: 181 | fat: 15g | protein: 6g | carbs: 9g | fiber: 5g

Spiced Sorghum and Berries

Prep time: 5 minutes | Cook time: about 1 hour | Serves 4

1 cup whole-grain sorghum
1 teaspoon ground cinnamon
1 teaspoon Chinese five-spice powder
3 cups water, plus more as needed
1 cup unsweetened nondairy milk
1 teaspoon vanilla extract
2 tablespoons pure maple syrup (optional)
1 tablespoon chia seeds
¼ cup sliced almonds
2 cups fresh raspberries, divided

1. In a large pot over medium-high heat, stir together the sorghum, cinnamon, five-spice powder, and water. Bring the water to a boil, cover the pot, and reduce the heat to medium-low. Cook for 1 hour, or until the sorghum is soft and chewy. If the sorghum grains are still hard, add another cup of water and cook for 15 minutes more. 2. In a glass measuring cup, whisk together the milk, vanilla, and maple syrup (if using) to blend. Add the mixture to the sorghum, along with the chia seeds, almonds, and 1 cup of raspberries. Gently stir to combine. 3. Serve topped with the remaining 1 cup of fresh raspberries.

Per Serving:
calories: 289 | fat: 8g | protein: 9g | carbs: 52g | fiber: 10g

Breakfast Hummus on Toast

Prep time: 10 minutes | Cook time: 1 hour | Serves 12

¼ cup vegetable broth
1 yellow onion, diced
1 garlic clove, minced
1 teaspoon ground cumin
1 teaspoon smoked paprika
½ teaspoon curry powder
½ teaspoon ground turmeric
¼ teaspoon black pepper, plus more to taste
1 sprig thyme
2 cups water
1 cup dried chickpeas, soaked overnight, drained, and rinsed
½ cup nutritional yeast
2 tablespoons tahini
1 tablespoon reduced-sodium tamari or red miso
Salt (optional)
Toast, for serving

1. Begin by heating a medium saucepan over medium heat. Add the broth to the pan. Sauté the onion, stirring often, until it becomes softened, which should take about 5 minutes. Add the garlic, cumin, paprika, curry powder, turmeric, ¼ teaspoon of pepper, and thyme. Cook for an additional 2 minutes. 2. Next, add water and chickpeas to the saucepan. Increase the heat to high and bring the mixture to a boil. Once boiling, reduce the heat to medium-low, cover the pan, and cook until the chickpeas are tender, approximately 45 minutes. 3. Drain the cooked chickpeas, but make sure to reserve the cooking water. Transfer the chickpeas to a food processor along with nutritional yeast, tahini, and tamari. Pulse the ingredients to combine, then continue to purée until a smooth consistency is achieved. Gradually add the reserved cooking liquid, one tablespoon at a time, until the desired consistency is reached. Keep in mind that the hummus will thicken slightly as it cools. 4. Season the hummus with salt (if desired) and additional pepper to taste. Serve the hummus on toast. It can be refrigerated for up to 5 days.

Per Serving:
calories: 104 | fat: 3g | protein: 6g | carbs: 14g | fiber: 3g

Spelt Berry Hot Breakfast Cereal

Prep time: 5 minutes | Cook time: 55 minutes | Serves 2

1 cup spelt berries
¼ teaspoon salt (optional)
⅛ teaspoon ground cinnamon
⅛ teaspoon ground cloves
2 cups unsweetened almond milk
¾ cup dates, pitted and chopped
¼ teaspoon orange zest

1. Bring 2½ cups of water to a boil in a medium saucepan. Add the spelt, salt (if using), cinnamon, and cloves. Cover the pot and bring the mixture to a boil. Reduce the heat to medium-low and cook for 45 to 50 minutes, or until the spelt is tender. Drain any excess water. 2. Add the almond milk, dates, and orange zest to the cooked spelt berries and simmer over medium-low heat for 10 to 12 minutes, or until heated through and creamy.

Per Serving:
calories: 423 | fat: 2g | protein: 18g | carbs: 88g | fiber: 13g

Vanilla Protein Pancakes

Prep time: 5 minutes | Cook time: 15 minutes | Serves 8

1½ cups pea protein isolate
½ cup whole wheat flour
1½ cups almond milk or water
2 teaspoons baking powder
2 teaspoons vanilla extract
Optional Toppings:
Walnuts
Fresh or frozen blueberries
Shredded coconut

1. Add all ingredients to a blender and blend until smooth, scraping down the sides of the blender to prevent any lumps if necessary. 2. Put a nonstick frying pan over medium heat. 3. Pour a large tablespoon of batter into the frying pan and bake until the edges are dry and bubbles form in the pancake. 4. Flip the pancake and bake the other side until it's lightly browned. 5. Repeat the process for the remaining pancake batter. 6. Serve the pancakes with the optional toppings and enjoy! 7. Store the pancakes in an airtight container in the fridge and consume within 3 days. Alternatively, store in the freezer for a maximum of 30 days and thaw at room temperature. Use a microwave or nonstick frying pan to reheat the pancakes before serving.

Per Serving:
calories: 120 | fat: 2g | protein: 18g | carbs: 9g | fiber: 2g

Avocado Toast

Prep time: 10 minutes | Cook time: 0 minutes | Makes 2 slices

1 ripe avocado, halved, pitted, and sliced
2 large slices toast
Salt (optional)

1. Mash the avocado in a small bowl and spread onto the toast. Sprinkle with salt, if desired.

Per Serving: (1 slice)
calories: 243 | fat: 16g | protein: 5g | carbs: 24g | fiber: 9g

Overnight Muesli

Prep time: 15 minutes | Cook time: 0 minutes | Serves 6

2 cups old-fashioned oats
1 cup raisins
½ cup wheat germ
½ cup oat bran
½ cup chopped dates
½ cup pepitas
¼ cup wheat bran
¼ cup slivered almonds
¼ cup chopped walnuts
¼ cup sunflower seed kernels
7 cups almond milk or other dairy-free milk

1. Place all the dry ingredients in a large mixing bowl. Mix well. Pour in the milk and mix well again. 2. Cover and place in the refrigerator to sit overnight. 3. The muesli is ready to eat in the morning and keeps for 4 to 5 days.

Per Serving:
calories: 423 | fat: 17g | protein: 16g | carbs: 46g | fiber: 11g

Ful Medames (Egyptian Breakfast Beans)

Prep time: 15 minutes | **Cook time:** 2 hours | **Serves 4**

1½ pounds (680 g) dried fava beans, soaked for 8 to 10 hours
1 medium yellow onion, peeled and diced small
4 cloves garlic, peeled and minced
1 teaspoon ground cumin
Zest and juice of 1 lemon
Salt, to taste (optional)
1 lemon, quartered

1. Start by draining and rinsing the beans. Place them in a large pot and add enough water to cover the beans by 4 inches. Bring the water to a boil over high heat, then reduce the heat to medium. Cover the pot and cook the beans for approximately 1½ to 2 hours, or until they are tender. 2. While the beans are cooking, take a medium skillet or saucepan and sauté the onion over medium heat for about 8 to 10 minutes. Cook until the onion becomes tender and starts to brown. Add the garlic, cumin, lemon zest, and lemon juice to the skillet. Cook for an additional 5 minutes. Set aside until the beans finish cooking. 3. Once the beans are fully cooked, drain most of the liquid from the pot, leaving about ½ cup behind. Add the onion mixture to the beans and mix well. Season with salt if desired. Serve the dish garnished with lemon quarters.

Per Serving:
calories: 170 | fat: 1g | protein: 14g | carbs: 35g | fiber: 13g

Red Flannel Beet Hash with Dill

Prep time: 15 minutes | **Cook time:** 55 minutes | **Serves 6**

2 medium Yukon gold potatoes, chopped into 1-inch pieces
2 medium beets, peeled and chopped into ½-inch pieces
1 tablespoon apple cider vinegar
2 tablespoons virgin olive oil (optional)
1 medium cooking onion, diced
1 teaspoon ground coriander
Salt and pepper, to taste (optional)
2 green onions, thinly sliced
¼ cup lightly packed chopped fresh dill
½ ripe avocado, peeled, pitted and chopped

1. Place the chopped potatoes and beets into a large saucepan or braiser-style pot. Cover the vegetables with cold water by 1 inch. Add the apple cider vinegar. Bring to a boil over medium-high heat. Lower the heat to a simmer and cook until the potatoes are tender and the beets are just tender, about 20 minutes. Drain the vegetables and set aside. 2. Heat the olive oil in a large skillet over medium heat. Add the onions and cook until lightly soft, about 3 minutes. Add the coriander, salt, if using, and pepper and stir until fragrant, about 30 seconds. 3. Add the drained potatoes and beets to the skillet and spread them out in a single layer. Let sit for 5 minutes before stirring. Flip and stir the hash every 5 minutes. Cook the hash for 20 minutes, or until the edges of the potatoes begin to crisp. 4. Lightly toss the hash with the green onions and dill. Serve the hash hot with chopped avocado on top.

Per Serving:
calories: 144 | fat: 7g | protein: 3g | carbs: 19g | fiber: 4g

Millet Porridge

Prep time: 5 minutes | **Cook time:** 25 minutes | **Makes 4 cups**

1 cup millet, soaked overnight in 2 cups filtered water
4 cups filtered water
Pinch of fine sea salt (optional)

1. Drain and thoroughly rinse the millet. Transfer it to an upright blender, add the 4 cups water and the salt, if using, and pulse until the grains are coarsely ground. Pour the mixture into a medium pot and bring to a boil over high heat, whisking frequently. Cover the pot, reduce the heat to low, and simmer for 18 to 20 minutes, stirring occasionally with a wooden spoon to prevent sticking, until the porridge is thick and creamy and no longer has a raw taste. 2. Serve hot. Pour leftover porridge into a widemouthed glass jar or other container and allow to cool, then cover tightly and store in the fridge for up to 5 days.

Per Serving: (1 cup)
calories: 189 | fat: 2g | protein: 6g | carbs: 36g | fiber: 4g

Cauliflower Scramble

Prep time: 15 minutes | **Cook time:** 15 minutes | **Serves 4**

1 yellow onion, diced
3 garlic cloves, minced
1 green bell pepper, seeded and coarsely chopped
1 red bell pepper, seeded and coarsely chopped
1 tablespoon water, plus more as needed
1 large cauliflower head, cored, florets coarsely chopped to about ½-inch dice
1 teaspoon ground turmeric
¼ cup nutritional yeast
¼ teaspoon ground nutmeg
¼ teaspoon cayenne pepper
¼ teaspoon freshly ground black pepper
1 tablespoon coconut aminos
1 (15-ounce /425-g) can chickpeas, drained and rinsed

1. In a large nonstick skillet over medium heat, combine the onion, garlic, and green and red bell peppers. Cook for 2 to 3 minutes, stirring, until the onion is translucent but not browned. Add the water, 1 tablespoon at a time, to avoid sticking or burning, as needed. 2. Add the cauliflower and toss to combine. Cover the skillet and cook for 5 to 6 minutes, or until the cauliflower is fork-tender. 3. In a small bowl, stir together the turmeric, nutritional yeast, nutmeg, cayenne pepper, and black pepper. Set aside. 4. Evenly sprinkle the coconut aminos over the cauliflower mixture and stir to combine. Stir in the spice mixture. Stir in the chickpeas and cook, uncovered, for 5 minutes to warm.

Per Serving:
calories: 243 | fat: 3g | protein: 18g | carbs: 40g | fiber: 14g

Eggplant Bacon

Prep time: 10 minutes | Cook time: 35 minutes | Serves 4

1 large eggplant
1 tablespoon sea salt (optional)
1 tablespoon virgin olive oil (optional)
1 tablespoon pure maple syrup (optional)
1 tablespoon apple cider vinegar
1 teaspoon smoked paprika
½ teaspoon gluten-free tamari soy sauce
½ teaspoon mellow or light miso
Freshly ground black pepper, to taste

1. Preheat the oven to 400ºF (205ºC). Set a cooling rack on top of a parchment-lined baking sheet. 2. Cut off both ends of the eggplant. Then, with the cut bottom end flat on the cutting board, cut the eggplant down the middle. Lay each half, cut side down, on the board, and slice into ¼-inch strips. 3. In a large colander, layer the eggplant strips, sprinkling liberally with sea salt as you go. After you finish the layering, let the eggplant sit for 15 minutes. 4. Rinse the eggplant thoroughly. Towel-dry the pieces of eggplant, and arrange them on the rack-fitted baking sheet. 5. In a small bowl, whisk together the olive oil, maple syrup, if using, apple cider vinegar, smoked paprika, tamari, and miso. Brush half of this mixture onto the eggplant strips. Season the eggplant with black pepper. 6. Slide the baking sheet into the oven and roast for 20 minutes. Remove the eggplant and use tongs to carefully flip over all the strips. Brush the remaining half of the oil and maple syrup mixture onto the exposed side of the eggplant. Season the eggplant with black pepper once more. Roast the eggplant for another 15 minutes or until you start seeing some crisped edges. Serve eggplant bacon hot.

Per Serving:
calories: 81 | fat: 4g | protein: 2g | carbs: 12g | fiber: 5g

Apple Cinnamon Oats Bowl

Prep time: 5 minutes | Cook time: 5 minutes | Serves 2

1 green apple, peeled and cored
1 cup instant oats
1 scoop soy protein isolate, chocolate flavor
¼ cup raisins
1 tablespoon cinnamon
2 cups water
Optional Toppings:
Apple slices
Raisins
Cinnamon

1. Cut the cored and peeled apple into tiny pieces and add them to a saucepan. 2. Add the water and oats to the saucepan and put it over medium heat. 3. Bring to a boil and cook the oats for about 5 minutes. 4. Turn the heat off, add the soy isolate, raisins and cinnamon, then stir thoroughly until everything is well combined. 5. Serve warm with the optional toppings and enjoy! 6. Store the oats in an airtight container in the fridge, and consume within 2 days. Alternatively, store in the freezer for a maximum of 60 days and thaw at room temperature.

Per Serving:
calories: 366 | fat: 4g | protein: 28g | carbs: 63g | fiber: 10g

Cleansing Morning Lemonade

Prep time: 2 minutes | Cook time: 0 minutes | Makes 1 quart

1 large lemon
1 quart warm purified water
Pinch of cayenne pepper, or to taste
1 to 2 teaspoons raw agave nectar (optional)

1. Thoroughly wash the lemon and extract its juice into a 1-quart glass or mason jar. Add purified water, cayenne pepper, and agave (if desired). 2. Stir the mixture well. Consume it first thing in the morning on an empty stomach.

Per Serving:
calories: 5 | fat: 0g | protein: 0g | carbs: 1g | fiber: 0g

Spring Breakfast Salad

Prep time: 5 minutes | Cook time: 0 minutes | Serves 2

½ cup strawberries
½ cup blueberries
½ cup blackberries
½ cup raspberries
1 grapefruit, peeled and segmented
3 tablespoons fresh orange juice (from 1 orange)
1 tablespoon pure maple syrup (optional)
¼ cup chopped fresh mint
¼ cup sliced almonds

1. Place the berries and grapefruit in a serving bowl. 2. In a small bowl, mix together the orange juice and maple syrup (if desired). Pour this syrup mixture over the fruit in the serving bowl. 3. Sprinkle the mint and almonds over the fruit. 4. Serve the fruit salad immediately.

Per Serving:
calories: 199 | fat: 6g | protein: 4g | carbs: 34g | fiber: 8g

Paradise Island Overnight Oatmeal

Prep time: 5 minutes | Cook time: 0 minutes | Serves 2

2 cups rolled oats
2 cups plant-based milk
½ cup fresh or frozen mango, diced
½ cup fresh or frozen pineapple chunks
1 sliced banana
1 tablespoon maple syrup (optional)
1 tablespoon chia seeds

1. Combine oats, milk, mango, pineapple, banana, maple syrup (if using), and chia seeds in a large bowl. 2. Cover the bowl and refrigerate the mixture overnight or for at least 4 hours before serving.

Per Serving:
calories: 510 | fat: 12g | protein: 14g | carbs: 93g | fiber: 15g

High-Protein Chocolate Blender Muffins

Prep time: 15 minutes | **Cook time:** 20 minutes | **Serves 6**

1 (15 ounces / 425 g) can black beans, drained and rinsed
½ cup applesauce
2 tablespoons ground chia seeds
¼ cup dairy-free milk
1 tablespoon lemon juice
½ cup maple syrup (optional)
2 teaspoons vanilla extract
1 tablespoon flaxseed
½ cup unsweetened cocoa powder
1 teaspoon baking powder
½ teaspoon baking soda
½ cup old-fashioned oats
½ cup dairy-free chocolate chips
¼ cup raw shelled hempseed

1. Preheat the oven to 350ºF (180ºC). 2. Line a twelve-cup muffin tin with paper liners. 3. Place all the ingredients in a blender except the chocolate chips and the hempseed. Blend until the mixture is as smooth as possible. Add the chocolate chips and hempseed and blend 5 seconds or until dispersed. 4. Pour into the muffin cups, filling at least three-quarters full. Bake for 20 minutes. Cool for 5 minutes, and then move the paper cups to a wire rack to cool completely. 5. Store in the refrigerator for up to 3 days or freeze up to 6 months.

Per Serving: (2 muffins)
calories: 174 | fat: 4g | protein: g | carbs: 27g | fiber: 6g

Shiitake Bakin'

Prep time: 5 minutes | **Cook time:** 30 minutes | **Makes 1 cup**

1 (3½ ounces / 99 g) package shiitake mushrooms, stems discarded and sliced thinly
1 teaspoon maple syrup (optional)
1 teaspoon reduced-sodium, gluten-free tamari
¼ teaspoon black pepper
¼ teaspoon garlic powder
¼ teaspoon smoked paprika

1. Preheat the oven to 375ºF (190ºC). Line a baking sheet with parchment paper. 2. Combine the shiitakes, maple syrup (if desired), tamari, pepper, garlic powder, and paprika in a medium bowl. 3. Spread the mushrooms in a single layer and bake for 30 minutes, tossing every 10 minutes, until the mushrooms start to crisp. Remove from the oven and allow to cool on the baking sheet before serving. The mushrooms can be stored in an airtight container for up to 3 days.

Per Serving: (1 cup)
calories: 55 | fat: 1g | protein: 2g | carbs: 10g | fiber: 1g

Zucchini Bread Oatmeal

Prep time: 5 minutes | **Cook time:** 20 minutes | **Serves 4**

2 cups rolled oats
1 medium zucchini, grated
4 cups water
½ cup unsweetened plant-based milk
1 tablespoon ground cinnamon
½ cup raisins
1 tablespoon maple syrup (optional)
Pinch of salt (optional)
2 medium bananas, sliced
4 tablespoons chopped walnuts (optional)

1. In a medium saucepan over medium-high, combine the oats, zucchini, and water and bring to a boil. Lower the heat to medium-low and simmer, stirring often, until the oats are soft and creamy, about 15 minutes. Remove from the heat, add the plant-based milk, cinnamon, raisins, maple syrup, and salt (if using) and stir well. 2. Divide the oatmeal among 4 bowls and top each portion with ½ sliced banana and 1 tablespoon of walnuts (if using).

Per Serving:
calories: 301 | fat: 4g | protein: 9g | carbs: 62g | fiber: 8g

Vanilla Buckwheat Porridge

Prep time: 5 minutes | **Cook time:** 25 minutes | **Serves 4**

3 cups water
1 cup raw buckwheat groats
1 teaspoon ground cinnamon
1 banana, sliced
¼ cup golden raisins
¼ cup dried currants
¼ cup sunflower seeds
2 tablespoons chia seeds
1 tablespoon hemp seeds
1 tablespoon sesame seeds, toasted
½ cup unsweetened nondairy milk
1 tablespoon pure maple syrup (optional)
1 teaspoon vanilla extract

1. In an 8-quart pot over high heat, bring the water to a boil. Stir in the buckwheat, cinnamon, and banana. Bring the mixture to a boil, stirring, then reduce the heat to medium-low. Cover the pot and cook for 15 minutes, or until the buckwheat is tender. Remove from the heat. 2. Stir in the raisins, currants, sunflower seeds, chia seeds, hemp seeds, sesame seeds, milk, maple syrup (if using), and vanilla. Cover the pot and let sit for 10 minutes before serving. 3. Serve as is or top as desired.

Per Serving:
calories: 353 | fat: 11g | protein: 10g | carbs: 61g | fiber: 10g

Chapter 3
Basics

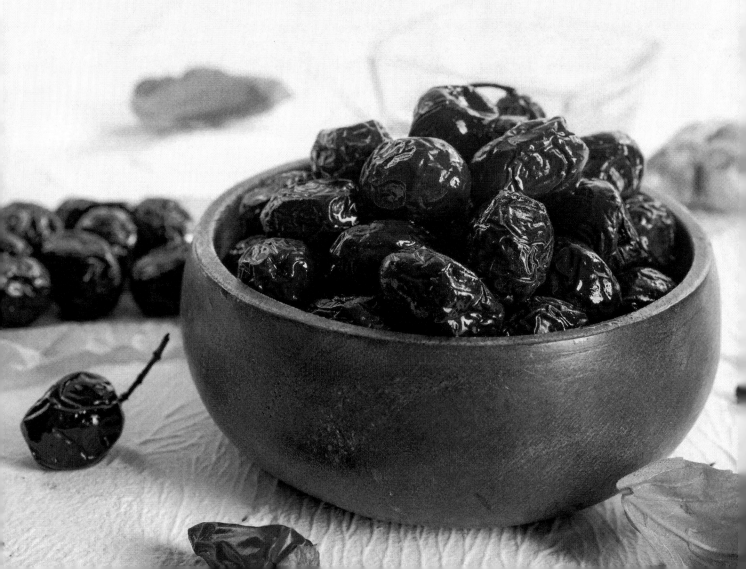

Herbed Millet Pizza Crust

Prep time: 5 minutes | Cook time: 40 minutes | Makes 1 large thin-crust pizza crust

½ cup coarsely ground millet
1½ cups water
1 tablespoon mixed dried Italian herbs
¼ teaspoon sea salt (optional)
1 to 2 tablespoons nutritional yeast

1. Preheat the oven to 350ºF (180ºC). Prepare an 8-inch-round pie dish or springform pan by lining it with parchment paper, allowing you to easily remove the crust once it's cooked. Using a nonstick pan is recommended to prevent sticking as the crust may be fragile until cooled. 2. In a small pot, combine millet, water, and a pinch of salt. Bring it to a boil, then cover and simmer for 15 to 20 minutes. Stir occasionally to prevent sticking. For a stronger flavor, you can add dried herbs while cooking the millet or stir them in after it's cooked. 3. Once the millet is cooked, add salt (if desired) and nutritional yeast. Spread the seasoned millet evenly in your prepared pan, ensuring it reaches the edges. 4. Place the crust in the oven for approximately 20 minutes or until the edges are lightly browned.

Per Serving: (1 crust)
calories: 378 | fat: 4g | protein: 11g | carbs: 72g | fiber: 8g

Cauliflower Béchamel

Prep time: 15 minutes | Cook time: 30 minutes | Makes about 3½ cups

1 large head cauliflower, cut into florets (about 3 cups)
Unsweetened plain almond milk, as needed
1 medium yellow onion, peeled and diced small
2 cloves garlic, peeled and minced
2 teaspoons minced thyme
¼ cup finely chopped basil
¼ cup nutritional yeast (optional)
¼ teaspoon ground nutmeg
Salt and freshly ground black pepper, to taste

1. In a large pot, add cauliflower and enough water to cover it. Bring to a boil over high heat and cook until the cauliflower becomes very tender, approximately 10 minutes. Drain any excess water and use an immersion blender or a blender with a tight-fitting lid (covered with a towel) to purée the cauliflower. If needed, add almond milk to achieve a creamy consistency. Set the purée aside while you prepare the remaining ingredients. 2. Place the onion in a large skillet or saucepan and sauté over medium heat for 10 minutes. To prevent sticking, add 1 to 2 tablespoons of water at a time. Add garlic, thyme, and basil, and cook for an additional minute. Stir in nutritional yeast (if using), nutmeg, salt, and pepper, and cook for 5 minutes or until heated through. 3. Combine the onion mixture with the cauliflower purée and blend until smooth. If necessary, add up to ½ cup of water to reach the desired smooth consistency.

Per Serving: (½ cup)
calories: 38 | fat: 0g | protein: 3g | carbs: 6g | fiber: 3g

Spicy Cilantro Pesto

Prep time: 10 minutes | Cook time: 0 minutes | Makes about 1 cup

2 cups packed cilantro
¼ cup hulled sunflower seeds, toasted (optional)
1 jalapeño pepper, coarsely chopped (for less heat, remove the seeds)
4 cloves garlic, peeled and chopped
Zest and juice of 1 lime
Salt, to taste (optional)
½ package extra-firm silken tofu (about 6 ounces / 170 g), drained
¼ cup nutritional yeast (optional)

1. In the bowl of a food processor, combine cilantro, sunflower seeds (if desired), jalapeño pepper, garlic, lime zest and juice, salt (if desired), tofu, and nutritional yeast (if desired). Process until the mixture is smooth and creamy.

Per Serving: (¼ cup)
calories: 143 | fat: 8g | protein: 11g | carbs: 10g | fiber: 5g

Pineapple Chutney

Prep time: 25 minutes | Cook time: 15 minutes | Makes 1½ cups

½ medium yellow onion, peeled and diced small
1 tablespoon grated ginger
2 jalapeño peppers, seeded and minced
½ tablespoon cumin seeds, toasted and ground
½ fresh pineapple, peeled, cored, and diced
½ cup finely chopped cilantro
Salt, to taste (optional)

1. In a large skillet or saucepan, place the onion and sauté over medium heat for 7 to 8 minutes. To prevent sticking, add 1 to 2 tablespoons of water at a time. 2. Add ginger, jalapeño peppers, and cumin seeds to the skillet and cook for an additional 4 minutes. Then, add pineapple and remove the pan from the heat. Stir in cilantro and salt (if desired).

Per Serving: (½ cup)
calories: 98 | fat: 0g | protein: 2g | carbs: 24g | fiber: 3g

Green Split Peas

Prep time: 5 minutes | Cook time: 45 minutes | Makes 2 cups

1 cup split peas, rinsed
1½ cups water

1. Place the split peas and water in a large pot with a lid. 2. Bring the mixture to a boil over high heat. 3. Once boiling, cover the pot with the lid and reduce the heat to low. 4. Allow the split peas to simmer for 45 minutes. 5. Transfer the cooked split peas to an airtight container and store them in the refrigerator for up to 5 days.

Per Serving: (1 cup)
calories: 347 | fat: 1g | protein: 24g | carbs: 63g | fiber: 25g

Quinoa

Prep time: 5 minutes | Cook time: 5 minutes | Makes 3 cups

1 cup quinoa

1½ cups vegetable broth

1. Place the quinoa in a fine-mesh strainer and rinse it under cold water. 2. Add the rinsed quinoa and broth to the pressure cooker. Cook on high pressure for 5 minutes. 3. Release the pressure, remove the lid, and fluff the quinoa with a fork. 4. Transfer the cooked quinoa to an airtight container and store it in the refrigerator for up to 5 days.

Per Serving: (1 cup)
calories: 214 | fat: 3g | protein: 8g | carbs: 38g | fiber: 4g

Tomato Sauce

Prep time: 10 minutes | Cook time: 40 minutes | Makes 4 cups

1 medium yellow onion, peeled and diced small
6 cloves garlic, peeled and minced
6 tablespoons minced basil
2 tablespoons minced oregano
1 (28-ounce / 794-g) can diced tomatoes, puréed
Salt, to taste (optional)

1. In a large saucepan, place the onion and sauté over medium heat for 10 minutes. To prevent sticking, add 1 to 2 tablespoons of water at a time. 2. Add garlic, basil, and oregano to the saucepan and cook for another 3 minutes. Then, add the puréed tomatoes and salt (if desired). Cover the saucepan and simmer over medium-low heat for 25 minutes.

Per Serving: (1 cup)
calories: 48 | fat: 0g | protein: 2g | carbs: 10g | fiber: 4g

Gut-Healing Sauerkraut

Prep time: 5 minutes | Cook time: 0 minutes | Makes 4 cups

1 medium purple cabbage
1 tablespoon Celtic sea salt (optional)
2 to 4 tablespoons minced fresh ginger, to taste (optional)

1. Begin by removing any wrinkly, dry, or damaged outer leaves from the cabbage and discarding them. Set aside one healthy and pliable leaf for later use. Cut the cabbage into quarters, making sure to cut through the core. Carefully remove and discard the tough inner core. Shred the cabbage using a mandoline, knife, or food processor. We recommend using a food processor with a shredding blade. 2. Place the shredded cabbage in a large bowl. Sprinkle salt (if desired) over the cabbage and massage it with your hands until liquid starts to release. Set the bowl aside to allow the cabbage to marinate. 3. Add minced ginger to the bowl of cabbage. Use your hands to evenly distribute the ginger throughout the cabbage, then continue massaging the cabbage until it releases a significant amount of liquid when squeezed. This liquid will serve as the brine. 4. Transfer the cabbage to a 1-quart mason jar with a wide mouth, packing it tightly with each handful added to the jar. Take the reserved cabbage leaf and gently fold it until it matches the width of the jar. Place the folded leaf on top of the packed cabbage, ensuring it covers the entire surface. 5. Press the cabbage leaf down firmly and pour enough brine from the mixing bowl to completely submerge the cabbage in the liquid. It is important that the cabbage remains below the water level to avoid exposure to oxygen. Leave about an inch of space between the top of the liquid and the top of the jar to allow for expansion. However, be cautious not to leave too much room as excessive oxygen could spoil the kraut.
6. Allow the kraut to ferment in a cool, dark place for a minimum of 3 days and up to 10 days, depending on your preferred level of sourness. Once the kraut has reached your desired taste, seal the jar and transfer it to the refrigerator. Fermentation will continue at a much slower pace in the fridge, and the flavors may continue to evolve over time.

Per Serving:
calories: 45 | fat: 0g | protein: 2g | carbs: 10g | fiber: 3g

Tahini Dressing

Prep time: 5 minutes | Cook time: 0 minutes | Makes ½ cup

¼ cup tahini
1 teaspoon minced garlic
3 tablespoons lemon juice
1 tablespoon maple syrup (optional)
1 teaspoon soy sauce
1 teaspoon ground cumin
1 tablespoon olive oil (optional)
1 tablespoon hot water
Pinch of salt and pepper (optional)

1. Combine all the ingredients in a small bowl and whisk until thoroughly mixed.
2. Transfer the mixture to an airtight container and store in the refrigerator for up to 7 days.

Per Serving: (½ cup)
calories: 283 | fat: 24g | protein: 6g | carbs: 16g | fiber: 3g

Cheesy Sprinkle

Prep time: 5 minutes | Cook time: 0 minutes | Makes ½ cup

½ cup ground sunflower seeds, or Brazil nuts, or macadamia nuts
2 teaspoons sea salt (optional)
1 to 2 tablespoons nutritional yeast
1 tablespoon olive oil (optional)

1. Place the sunflower seeds in a small bowl, then add the salt (if using) and nutritional yeast. Mix to combine. 2. Leave as is for a dry sprinkle, or add just enough olive oil (if using) to bring the mixture together into a crumbly texture.

Per Serving: (1 tablespoon)
calories: 284 | fat: 25g | protein: 9g | carbs: 9g | fiber: 4g

Creamy Avocado-Lime Dressing

Prep time: 5 minutes | **Cook time:** 0 minutes | **Serves 6**

1 avocado, diced	½ teaspoon ground cumin
¼ cup fresh lime or lemon juice	¼ teaspoon salt (optional)
¼ cup cilantro leaves	½ cup water, plus more as needed

1. In a high-speed blender, blend all the ingredients until a smooth consistency is achieved. Adjust the seasoning as desired. 2. Gradually add water, 1 tablespoon at a time, and continue blending until the desired consistency is reached. Add more water if needed. 3. Use the blended mixture within 1 day for optimal freshness.

Per Serving:
calories: 57 | fat: 5g | protein: 1g | carbs: 4g | fiber: 2g

Tempeh Bacon

Prep time: 5 minutes | **Cook time:** 10 minutes | **Serves 4**

2 tablespoons soy sauce	1 (8-ounce / 227-g) package tempeh
1 tablespoon water	
1 tablespoon maple syrup (optional)	1 tablespoon canola oil (optional)
½ tablespoon liquid smoke	

1. In a medium bowl, combine soy sauce, water, maple syrup (optional), and liquid smoke. Set the mixture aside. 2. Cut the tempeh block in half lengthwise and thinly slice it. 3. Heat oil (optional) in a large pan over high heat. Add the tempeh slices in a single layer and cook for 2 minutes. Flip the slices and cook for an additional 2 minutes. 4. While the tempeh is still in the pan, pour in the liquid mixture. Sauté the tempeh for 3 minutes. Flip the slices and cook for another 3 minutes or until the liquid is absorbed. 5. For the best flavor and texture, serve the Tempeh Bacon immediately.

Per Serving:
calories: 17 | fat: 11g | protein: 11g | carbs: 11g | fiber: 0g

Plant-Based Fish Sauce

Prep time: 10 minutes | **Cook time:** 20 minutes | **Makes 3 to 4 cups**

4 cups water	¼ cup low-sodium soy sauce, tamari, or coconut aminos
1 (4-by-8-inch) sheet of kombu	3 garlic cloves, crushed
½ cup dried shiitake mushrooms	2 teaspoons rice vinegar

1. In a medium saucepan, combine water, kombu, mushrooms, soy sauce, garlic, and vinegar. Bring the mixture to a boil, then reduce the heat to low. 2. Cover the saucepan and let it simmer for 15 to 20 minutes. Remove from heat and keep it covered. Allow the mixture to steep overnight or for at least 8 hours. 3. Strain the liquid to remove any solids and discard them. Transfer the plant-based fish sauce to a glass bottle and store it in the refrigerator for up to 3 weeks. Remember to shake well before each use.

Per Serving:
calories: 4 | fat: 0g | protein: 0g | carbs: 1g | fiber: 0g

20-Minute Cashew Cheese Sauce

Prep time: 5 minutes | **Cook time:** 15 minutes | **Makes about 3 cups**

½ cup raw cashews	1 tablespoon lemon juice
1 cup peeled and diced potatoes	1 teaspoon miso paste
	½ teaspoon garlic powder
¼ cup diced carrots	½ teaspoon dry mustard
¼ cup diced onions	Pinch paprika
3 cups water	Ground black pepper
4 tablespoons nutritional yeast	Salt (optional)

1. Soak the cashews for 30 to 60 minutes in very hot (boiled) water before use in order for your sauce to be creamy and delicious. You can omit this step if you have a high-speed blender. 2. In a medium pot, combine the potatoes, carrots, and onion and cover with the water. Bring to a boil and cook for about 15 minutes, until the vegetables are tender and easily mushed with a fork. 3. While the vegetables are boiling, drain the cashews if you soaked them. Transfer them to a blender or food processor and add the nutritional yeast, lemon juice, miso paste, garlic powder, mustard, and paprika. Season with pepper and salt (if using). 4. When the vegetables are cooked, reserve 1 cup of cooking water and add it to the blender along with the cooked vegetables. Blend for 30 to 60 seconds, until smooth. This will keep for up to 4 days in the refrigerator.

Per Serving:
calories: 55 | fat: 3g | protein: 3g | carbs: 6g | fiber: 1g

Salsa Verde

Prep time: 20 minutes | **Cook time:** 0 minutes | **Makes 3 cups**

1 pound (454 g) tomatillos (about 16 medium), husks removed, coarsely chopped	and tender stems
	4 cloves garlic, peeled and chopped
2 poblano peppers, roasted, peeled, and seeded	1 serrano chile, chopped (for less heat, remove the seeds)
6 green onions (green and white parts), chopped	Zest of 2 limes
2 cups chopped cilantro leaves	Salt, to taste (optional)

1. In a bowl of food processor, mix all ingredients and purée until smooth and creamy.

Per Serving: (1 cup)
calories: 97 | fat: 1g | protein: 3g | carbs: 20g | fiber: 6g

Mango-Orange Dressing

Prep time: 5 minutes | Cook time: 0 minutes | Serves 8

1 cup diced mango
½ cup orange juice
2 tablespoons fresh lime juice
2 tablespoons gluten-free rice vinegar
1 teaspoon coconut sugar (optional)
¼ teaspoon salt (optional)
2 tablespoons chopped cilantro

1. In a blender, combine mango, orange juice, lime juice, rice vinegar, sugar, and salt (if desired). Blend until the mixture is smooth. Stir in the cilantro. 2. Transfer the dressing to an airtight container and refrigerate for up to 2 days.

Per Serving:
calories: 23 | fat: 0g | protein: 0g | carbs: 6g | fiber: 0g

Croutons

Prep time: 5 minutes | Cook time: 15 minutes | Serves 4

½ day-old baguette, sliced
2 tablespoons olive oil (optional)
½ tablespoon garlic salt (optional)

1. Preheat the oven to 350ºF (180ºC). 2. Brush olive oil onto the baguette slices and sprinkle with garlic salt, if desired. 3. Cut the bread into cubes, place them on a baking sheet, and bake for 10 to 15 minutes, or until they turn golden brown. 4. Let the croutons cool before serving. 5. For the best taste and texture, enjoy the croutons immediately after baking.

Per Serving:
calories: 94 | fat: 7g | protein: 1g | carbs: 7g | fiber: 0g

Pure Nut Mylk

Prep time: 2 minutes | Cook time: 0 minutes | Makes 3 cups

1 cup raw, unsalted nuts (almonds, hazelnuts, Brazil nuts, pecans, macadamias, walnuts)
3 cups purified water for blending, plus more if desired

1. Soak the nuts overnight in 2 to 3 cups of water. 2. Drain and discard the soaking water and rinse the nuts well. Place the nuts in a blender along with the 3 cups of purified water. Blend on high speed for 2 to 3 minutes, or until smooth. 3. Strain the blended nut mixture through a cheesecloth or a nut milk bag, squeezing out as much liquid as possible. 4. If you want a thinner nut mylk, add more purified water as desired. 5. Pour into a glass jar and refrigerate. The mylk will keep in the refrigerator for 3 to 4 days.

Per Serving:
calories: 276 | fat: 23g | protein: 10g | carbs: 10g | fiber: 6g

Hemp Mylk

Prep time: 5 minutes | Cook time: 0 minutes | Makes 3 cups

½ cup hemp hearts
3 cups purified water, for blending
½ teaspoon ground cinnamon
2 dates, pitted

1. Place all the ingredients in a blender and blend until smooth and creamy. 2. Transfer the hemp mylk to a glass jar with a tight lid and refrigerate. It will stay fresh for up to 5 days in the fridge.

Per Serving:
calories: 47 | fat: 0g | protein: 1g | carbs: 11g | fiber: 1g

Maple-Dijon Dressing

Prep time: 5 minutes | Cook time: 0 minutes | Serves 4

¼ cup apple cider vinegar
2 tablespoons maple syrup
2 teaspoons gluten-free Dijon mustard
¼ teaspoon black pepper
2 tablespoons water
Salt (optional)

1. Combine the vinegar, maple syrup (if desired), mustard, pepper and water in a small jar with a tight-fitting lid. Season with salt to taste, if desired. Refrigerate for up to 5 days.

Per Serving:
calories: 31 | fat: 0g | protein: 0g | carbs: 7g | fiber: 0g

Not-So-Fat Guacamole

Prep time: 15 minutes | Cook time: 13 minutes | Makes 2 cups

1 cup shelled edamame
1 cup broccoli florets
Zest of 1 lime and juice of 2 limes
2 Roma tomatoes, diced
½ small red onion, peeled and diced small
¼ cup finely chopped cilantro
1 clove garlic, peeled and minced (about 1 teaspoon)
Salt, to taste (optional)
1 pinch cayenne pepper, or to taste

1. Place the edamame in a medium saucepan and add water to cover. Bring to a boil and cook for 5 minutes. Drain and rinse the edamame until cooled. 2. Steam the broccoli in a double boiler or steamer basket for about 8 minutes, or until very tender. Drain and rinse the broccoli until cooled. 3. Add the edamame and broccoli to a food processor and purée until smooth and creamy. Add water if needed to achieve a creamy texture. Put the puréed mixture into a bowl and add the lime zest and juice, tomatoes, onion, cilantro, garlic, salt (if using), and cayenne. Mix well and chill until ready to serve.

Per Serving: (1 cup)
calories: 136 | fat: 4g | protein: 10g | carbs: 17g | fiber: 6g

Mama Mia Marinara Sauce

Prep time: 10 minutes | Cook time: 2 to 3 hours | Makes about 7 cups

1 medium onion, diced
5 garlic cloves, minced
2 (28-ounce / 794-g) cans no-salt-added crushed tomatoes
½ cup red wine
2 tablespoons Italian seasoning, or 1 tablespoon each dried basil and dried oregano
Ground black pepper
Salt (optional)

1. Put the onion, garlic, and tomatoes in the slow cooker. Swirl the wine in the empty tomato cans and pour everything into the slow cooker. Add the Italian seasoning, pepper, and salt (if using). Stir to combine. 2. Cover and cook on High for 2 to 3 hours or on Low for 4 to 5 hours.

Per Serving:
calories: 30 | fat: 0g | protein: 1g | carbs: 4g | fiber: 1g

Lemon-Thyme Dressing

Prep time: 5 minutes | Cook time: 0 minutes | Serves 6

⅓ cup fresh lemon juice
2 sprigs fresh thyme, leaves stripped and chopped, stems discarded
1 garlic clove, sliced in half
1 teaspoon gluten-free tahini
½ teaspoon coconut sugar (optional)
½ teaspoon salt (optional)
Pinch black pepper
¼ cup plain gluten-free hummus

1. Combine the lemon juice, thyme, garlic, tahini, sugar, salt (if desired), and pepper in a jar with a tight-fitting lid. Add the hummus in a slow, steady stream and adjust the seasoning. Refrigerate for up to 5 days. (Remove the garlic clove before serving.)

Per Serving:
calories: 7 | fat: 0g | protein: 0g | carbs: 2g | fiber: 0g

Buckwheat Sesame Milk

Prep time: 5 minutes | Cook time: 0 minutes | Makes 4 cups

1 cup cooked buckwheat
1 tablespoon tahini, or other nut or seed butter
1 teaspoon pure vanilla extract (optional)
2 to 3 dates, or 15 drops pure stevia (or vanilla stevia), or 2 to 3 tablespoons unrefined sugar (optional)
3 cups water

1. Put everything in a blender, and purée until smooth. 2. Strain the fiber through a piece of cheesecloth or a fine-mesh sieve. 3. Keep in an airtight container in the fridge for up to 5 days.

Per Serving: (1 cup)
calories: 76 | fat: 2g | protein: 2g | carbs: 12g | fiber: 1g

Greener Guacamole

Prep time: 15 minutes | Cook time: 0 minutes | Makes 1 to 1½ cups

2 ripe avocados, pitted, peeled, and diced
Juice of ½ lime
2 scallions, green and white parts, chopped
1 garlic clove, minced
½ teaspoon ground cumin
½ small bunch cilantro, chopped
Ground black pepper
Salt (optional)

1. In a medium bowl, mix together avocados, lime juice, scallions, garlic, cumin, cilantro, pepper, and salt (if desired). Mash the ingredients together using a fork until you reach your desired consistency. 2. Transfer the mixture to a serving bowl and refrigerate until ready to serve.

Per Serving:
calories: 40 | fat: 4g | protein: 1g | carbs: 3g | fiber: 2g

Oil-Free Hummus

Prep time: 10 minutes | Cook time: 0 minutes | Makes about 2 cups

1 (15-ounce / 425-g) can chickpeas, undrained
¼ cup raw sesame seeds
4 garlic cloves
Juice from ½ lemon
¾ teaspoon ground cumin
¼ teaspoon paprika
½ teaspoon salt (optional)

1. Put the chickpeas and about half of the liquid from the can in a blender or food processor. Add the sesame seeds, garlic, lemon juice, cumin, paprika, and salt (if using). Blend until creamy. Store in the refrigerator for up to 3 days.

Per Serving:
calories: 40 | fat: 2g | protein: 2g | carbs: 4g | fiber: 1g

Peanut Milk

Prep time: 5 minutes | Cook time: 0 minutes | Makes 3 cups

1 cup unsalted roasted peanuts
¼ cup raisins
3 cups water

1. In a blender pitcher, soak the peanuts and raisins in the water. Let the mixture sit overnight or for at least 6 hours. 2. Blend the water, peanuts, and raisins together on high for 1 to 2 minutes. 3. Using cheesecloth or a mesh nut-milk bag, strain the milk into a pitcher, separating out the liquid from the solids. 4. Store in an airtight container in the fridge for up to 5 days.

Per Serving: (1 cup)
calories: 284 | fat: 24g | protein: 14g | carbs: 9g | fiber: 4g

Fresh Tomato Salsa

Prep time: 15 minutes | Cook time: 0 minutes | Makes about 4 cups

3 large ripe tomatoes, diced small
1 small red onion, peeled and diced small
½ cup chopped cilantro
1 to 2 jalapeño peppers, minced (for less heat, remove the seeds)
2 cloves garlic, peeled and minced
3 tablespoons fresh lime juice
Salt, to taste (optional)

1. Combine all ingredients in a large bowl and mix well. Store refrigerated until ready to serve.

Per Serving: (1 cup)
calories: 38 | fat: 0g | protein: 1g | carbs: 8g | fiber: 2g

Strawberry Dressing

Prep time: 5 minutes | Cook time: 0 minutes | Makes 1½ cups

1½ cups chopped fresh strawberries
1 to 2 tablespoons agave, or maple syrup (optional)
½ tablespoon lemon juice

1. In a food processor or blender, blend all the ingredients until smooth. 2. Store in an airtight container in the fridge for up to 7 days.

Per Serving: (1 cup)
calories: 51 | fat: 0g | protein: 1g | carbs: 13g | fiber: 2g

Tofu Sour Cream

Prep time: 5 minutes | Cook time: 0 minutes | Makes 1½ cups

1 (12-ounce / 340-g) package extra-firm silken tofu, drained
1 tablespoon fresh lemon juice
1 tablespoon red wine vinegar
Salt, to taste (optional)

In a blender, mix all ingredients and purée until smooth and creamy. Chill until ready to serve.

Per Serving: (½ cup)
calories: 105 | fat: 6g | protein: 11g | carbs: 2g | fiber: 0g

Chapter 4: Beans and Grains

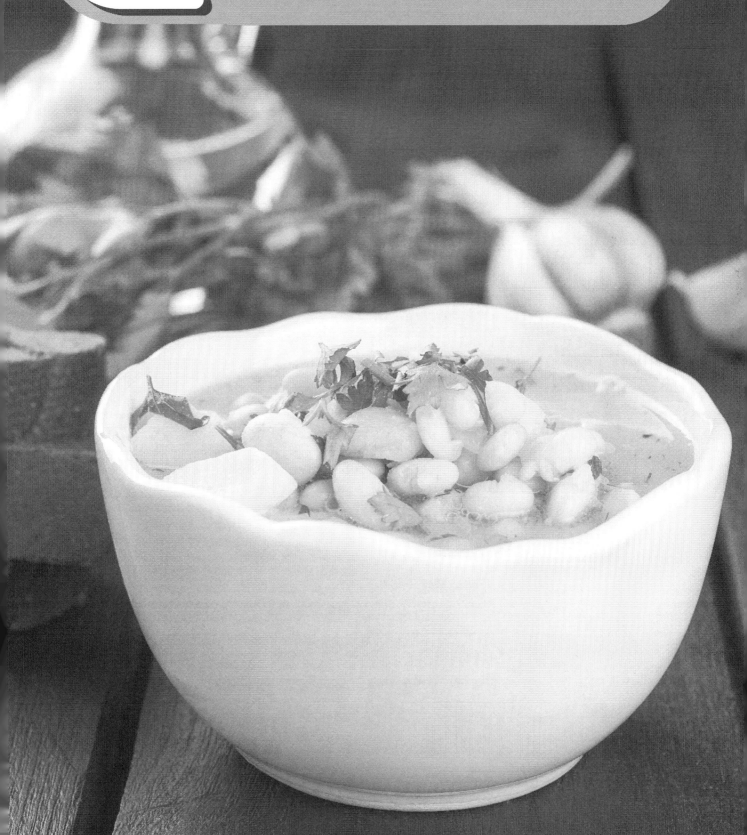

Lucky Black-Eyed Pea Stew

Prep time: 15 minutes | Cook time: 40 minutes | Serves 4

½ cup black-eyed peas, soaked
1 large carrot, peeled and cut into ½-inch pieces (about ¾ cup)
1 large beet, peeled and cut into ½-inch pieces (about ¾ cup)
¼ cup finely chopped parsley
¼ teaspoon cumin seeds, toasted and ground
¼ teaspoon turmeric
¼ teaspoon cayenne pepper
⅛ teaspoon asafetida
¼ teaspoon salt, or to taste (optional)
½ teaspoon fresh lime juice

1. In a pot, combine black-eyed peas and 3 cups of water. Cook over medium heat for 20 to 25 minutes. Add carrot and beet and cook for an additional 10 minutes. If the stew becomes too thick, add more water as needed. Stir in parsley, cumin, turmeric, cayenne pepper, and asafetida. Cook for another 5 to 7 minutes. Season with salt if desired. 2. Remove the pot from heat and stir in lime juice.

Per Serving:
calories: 106 | fat: 0g | protein: 6g | carbs: 19g | fiber: 7g

Quinoa Primavera

Prep time: 20 minutes | Cook time: 15 minutes | Serves 6

Citrus-Pickled Shallots:
2 large shallots, sliced in half, then into half-moons
2 tablespoons orange juice
½ teaspoon apple cider vinegar
½ teaspoon salt (optional)
Pinch of sugar (optional)
Quinoa:
2 cups water
1 cup quinoa, soaked at least 2 hours, rinsed, and drained
2 cups frozen artichoke hearts
2 garlic cloves, minced
1 teaspoon dried tarragon
½ teaspoon dried thyme
½ teaspoon salt, plus more to taste (optional)
¼ teaspoon dried dill
¼ teaspoon black pepper, plus more to taste
2 cups frozen peas
2 carrots, diced
1 orange or yellow bell pepper, chopped fine
3 scallions, sliced thin
Grated zest and juice of 1 lemon
½ cup raw sunflower seeds

1. In a small bowl, combine all the ingredients for the shallots. Refrigerate until ready to serve. The shallots can be kept in the fridge for up to 3 days. 2. To prepare the quinoa, combine water and quinoa in a large saucepan over high heat. Bring it to a boil, then add artichokes, garlic, tarragon, thyme, ½ teaspoon of salt (if desired), dill, and ¼ teaspoon of pepper. Reduce the heat to medium-low, cover the saucepan, and cook for 10 minutes. Then, reduce the heat to low and stir in peas, carrots, bell pepper, and scallions. Cover and continue cooking until the vegetables are heated through, approximately 5 minutes. 3. Remove the saucepan from the heat and add lemon juice, lemon zest, and sunflower seeds. Fluff the quinoa with a fork and season with salt and pepper to taste. Serve the quinoa, topping each portion with the prepared shallots. Leftovers can also be served cold.

Per Serving:
calories: 247 | fat: 8g | protein: 11g | carbs: 36g | fiber: 9g

Chickpea Pâté

Prep time: 10 minutes | Cook time: 0 minutes | Serves 4

1 cup whole raw nuts, toasted
2 tablespoons extra-virgin olive oil, plus more for drizzling (optional)
1 (15½-ounce / 439-g) can chickpeas, drained and rinsed well
½ cup filtered water
1 teaspoon fine sea salt, plus more to taste (optional)
½ teaspoon grated or pressed garlic
½ teaspoon raw apple cider vinegar

1. Place the nuts and oil in a food processor and blend until smooth, scraping down the sides as needed. This may take a few minutes to achieve a runny consistency. Add chickpeas, water, salt (if desired), garlic, and vinegar to the mixture. Blend until completely smooth, adding more cooking liquid or water if needed to reach the desired consistency. This process may take a couple of minutes. Adjust the salt to taste. 2. Serve the creamy mixture drizzled with olive oil, or store it in an airtight container in the refrigerator for up to 4 days.

Per Serving:
calories: 321 | fat: 22g | protein: 11g | carbs: 23g | fiber: 7g

Red Lentil Pâté

Prep time: 10 minutes | Cook time: 20 minutes | Serves 4

1 cup red lentils
1½ cups filtered water
1 (2-inch) piece kombu
3 large garlic cloves
3 tablespoons extra-virgin olive oil, plus more for serving (optional)
½ teaspoon fine sea salt, or to taste (optional)

1. Place the lentils in a medium-sized pot, cover them with tap water, gently swish them around using your fingers, and then drain the water. Repeat this process once more before returning the drained lentils back to the pot. Add filtered water, kombu, and garlic to the pot, and bring it to a boil over high heat. Once boiling, cover the pot, reduce the heat to low, and let it simmer for about 20 minutes, or until the lentils become soft and all the water has been absorbed. Remove the pot from the heat and take out the kombu (dispose of it properly, such as composting). 2. Add olive oil and salt (if desired) to the pot, and vigorously stir until the lentils and garlic become smooth and creamy. Drizzle some olive oil on top and serve the lentils warm or at room temperature. If there are any leftovers, store the cooled pâté in a jar or an airtight container in the refrigerator for up to 4 days.

Per Serving:
calories: 273 | fat: 11g | protein: 12g | carbs: 37g | fiber: 6g

Nut-Crusted Tofu

Prep time: 10 minutes | Cook time: 20 minutes | Makes 8 slices

- ½ cup roasted, shelled pistachios
- ¼ cup whole wheat bread crumbs
- 1 shallot, minced
- 1 garlic clove, minced
- 1 teaspoon grated lemon zest
- ½ teaspoon dried tarragon
- Salt and black pepper (optional)
- 1 (16-ounce / 454-g) package sprouted or extra-firm tofu, drained and sliced lengthwise into 8 pieces
- 1 tablespoon Dijon mustard
- 1 tablespoon lemon juice

1. Preheat your oven to 375ºF (190ºC) and line a baking sheet with parchment paper. 2. Using a food processor or a knife, chop the pistachios until they are roughly the size of bread crumbs. In a pie plate, combine the chopped pistachios, bread crumbs, shallot, garlic, lemon zest, and tarragon. Season the mixture with salt (if desired) and pepper. 3. Season the tofu slices with salt and pepper. In a small bowl, mix together the mustard and lemon juice. 4. Spread the mustard mixture evenly over the top and sides of each tofu slice. Press each slice into the bread crumb mixture, ensuring they are well coated. 5. Place the tofu slices on the prepared baking sheet with the uncoated side facing down. Sprinkle any remaining bread crumb mixture evenly on top of the slices. Bake in the preheated oven for about 20 minutes or until the tops are nicely browned. Serve and enjoy.

Per Serving: (1 slice)

calories: 114 | fat: 7g | protein: 8g | carbs: 7g | fiber: 1g

Mango Satay Tempeh Bowl

Prep time: 10 minutes | Cook time: 30 minutes | Serves 4

- 1 cup cooked or canned black beans
- ½ cup dry quinoa
- 1 (14-ounce / 397-g) pack tempeh, sliced
- 1 cup peanut butter
- 1 cup fresh or frozen mango cubes
- Optional Toppings:
- Chili flakes
- Shredded coconut

1. If using dry beans, soak and cook ⅓ cup of black beans as needed. Also, cook the quinoa for about 15 minutes until tender. 2. Blend the mango in a blender or food processor until smooth. Set aside. 3. Place tempeh slices and peanut butter in an airtight container. 4. Close the lid tightly and shake well to evenly coat the tempeh slices with peanut butter. 5. Preheat the oven to 375ºF (190ºC) and line a baking sheet with parchment paper. 6. Arrange the peanut butter-coated tempeh slices on the baking sheet and bake for approximately 15 minutes, or until the tempeh turns brown and crispy. 7. Divide the cooked black beans, quinoa, mango purée, and tempeh slices into two bowls. Optional toppings can be added according to preference. Enjoy! 8. Store any remaining mango tempeh bowl in an airtight container in the refrigerator and consume within 2 days. Alternatively, it can be stored in the freezer for up to 30 days. Thaw at room temperature before serving. It can be enjoyed cold, and reheating is not necessary for the tempeh and beans.

Per Serving:

calories: 536 | fat: 24g | protein: 30g | carbs: 55g | fiber: 7g

Tahini Green Beans

Prep time: 10 minutes | Cook time: 10 minutes | Serves 4

- 1 pound (454 g) green beans, washed and trimmed
- 2 tablespoons gluten-free tahini
- 1 minced garlic clove
- Grated zest and juice of 1 lemon
- Salt and black pepper (optional)
- 1 teaspoon toasted black or white sesame seeds (optional)

1. In a medium saucepan fitted with a steamer insert, steam the beans over medium-high heat. Once cooked, drain the beans and set aside, keeping the cooking water. 2. In a mixing bowl, combine tahini, garlic, lemon zest, lemon juice, salt (if desired), and pepper to taste. Use the reserved cooking water to thin the sauce to your preferred consistency. 3. Toss the steamed green beans with the sauce and serve them warm or at room temperature. If desired, garnish with sesame seeds.

Per Serving:

calories: 73 | fat: 5g | protein: 3g | carbs: 8g | fiber: 3g

Chorizo Chickpea Bowl

Prep time: 10 minutes | Cook time: 10 minutes | Serves 4

- 2 cups cooked or canned chickpeas
- 1 cup fresh or frozen spinach
- ¼ cup raisins
- ½ cup raw and unsalted cashews
- 2 tablespoons Mexican chorizo seasoning
- ½ cup water
- Optional Toppings:
- Raisins
- Parsley
- Lime juice

1. When using dry chickpeas, soak and cook ⅔ cup of dry chickpeas. 2. Put a nonstick deep frying pan over medium-high heat and add the spinach, chorizo seasoning and the water. 3. Stir continuously until everything is cooked, then add the chickpeas and cashew nuts. Make sure to stir again to mix everything. 4. Let it cook for about 10 minutes while stirring occasionally. 5. Turn the heat off, then add the raisins, stir well and drain the excess water. 6. Divide between 2 bowls, garnish with the optional toppings, serve and enjoy! 7. Store the chorizo chickpeas in an airtight container in the fridge, and consume within 2 days. Alternatively, store in the freezer for a maximum of 30 days and thaw at room temperature. The chorizo chickpeas can be eaten cold or reheated in a saucepan or a microwave.

Per Serving:

calories: 307 | fat: 10g | protein: 14g | carbs: 41g | fiber: 11g

Orzo "Risotto"

Prep time: 10 minutes | Cook time: 15 minutes | Serves 6

4 cups vegetable broth
1 tablespoon olive oil (optional)
1 large shallot or ¼ yellow onion, minced
1 teaspoon dried tarragon or dill
1 pound (454 g) whole wheat orzo
½ cup white wine
Grated zest and juice of 1 lemon
Salt and black pepper (optional)
Chopped flat-leaf parsley (optional)

1. In a medium saucepan, bring the broth to a boil. Reduce the heat to medium-low, cover the saucepan, and let it simmer. 2. Place a large saucepan over medium heat. If desired, add oil to the pan, followed by the shallot. Cover the pan and cook, stirring often, until the shallot becomes soft and translucent, which usually takes about 5 minutes. Stir in the tarragon and then add the orzo. 3. Pour in the wine and stir the orzo constantly until the wine is absorbed. 4. While stirring continuously, add the broth to the orzo, one cup at a time. The orzo will absorb the broth, resulting in a creamy texture. This process usually takes around 3 to 5 minutes. Repeat this step with the remaining broth. 5. Remove the saucepan from the heat. Stir in the lemon zest and juice, and season with salt (if desired) and pepper. If desired, garnish with parsley. Serve and enjoy.

Per Serving:
calories: 310 | fat: 4g | protein: 8g | carbs: 62g | fiber: 11g

Chickpea Tortilla Fajita Stack

Prep time: 20 minutes | Cook time: 0 minutes | Serves 4

Chickpea Tortillas:
1 tablespoon ground chia seeds
1 cup chickpea flour
¼ teaspoon sea salt (optional)
½ teaspoon ground cumin
2 tablespoons extra virgin olive oil (optional)
Filling:
1 tablespoon extra virgin olive oil (optional)
½ cup diced white onion
1 yellow bell pepper, diced
8 ounces (227 g) white mushrooms, diced
½ cup diced tomatoes
2 teaspoons fajita seasoning
½ teaspoon salt (optional)
¼ teaspoon ground black pepper
1 (15 ounces / 425 g) can pinto beans, drained and rinsed
2 tablespoons raw shelled hempseed
Salsa, for garnish
Avocado, for garnish

Make Chickpea Tortillas:

1. In a small bowl, mix ground chia seeds with 3 tablespoons of water. Set aside to thicken. 2. In a medium bowl, combine 1 cup of water, chickpea flour, chia seed mixture, salt (if desired), and cumin. 3. Stir the ingredients together until just combined. 4. Heat 2 tablespoons of oil (if desired) in an 8-inch skillet over medium-high heat. 5. Pour ¼ cup of the chickpea batter into the skillet and tilt the pan in a circular motion to spread the batter evenly, similar to making crepes. 6. Cook the tortilla until golden brown on one side, then flip and cook for another minute. Transfer to a plate. Repeat this process with the remaining batter until all the tortillas are made.

Make Filling:

7. Heat oil (if desired) in a large skillet over medium-high heat. Add onion, bell pepper, and mushrooms, and sauté for 10 to 15 minutes, or until the onion becomes translucent. Add tomatoes, fajita seasoning, salt (if desired), and pepper. Cook for an additional 5 minutes. Stir in the beans and hemp seeds, and heat through.

Assemble:

8. To assemble, start by placing one chickpea tortilla on a plate. Spoon about ½ cup of the filling onto the tortilla. Repeat this layering process with another tortilla and more filling until all the filling is used. Finish with a final tortilla on top. Top with salsa and avocado. Cut the stacked tortillas into quarters in a pie shape and serve.

Per Serving:
calories: 358 | fat: 12g | protein: 17g | carbs: 48g | fiber: 11g

Lentil-Mushroom No-Meat Pasta (Bolognese)

Prep time: 15 minutes | Cook time: 45 minutes | Serves 4

¼ cup mushroom stock
1 large yellow onion, finely diced
1 (10-ounce / 283-g) package cremini mushrooms, trimmed and chopped fine
2 tablespoons tomato paste
3 chopped garlic cloves
1 teaspoon oregano
2½ cups water
1 cup brown lentils
1 (28-ounce / 794-g) can puréed or diced tomatoes with basil
1 tablespoon balsamic vinegar
Pasta
Salt and black pepper (optional)
Chopped basil

1. Heat a large stockpot over medium heat and add the stock. Once the broth starts to simmer, add the onion and mushrooms. Cover the pot and cook for approximately 5 minutes until both vegetables are soft. Stir in the tomato paste, garlic, and oregano, and continue cooking for an additional 2 minutes while stirring constantly. 2. Add water and lentils to the pot. Bring it to a boil, then reduce the heat to medium-low and cover. Cook for 5 minutes. Stir in the tomatoes and vinegar. Replace the lid, reduce the heat to low, and continue cooking until the lentils become tender, which usually takes about 30 minutes. 3. In the meantime, cook the pasta according to the package instructions. 4. Remove the sauce from the heat and season with salt (if desired) and pepper to taste. Garnish with basil and serve the sauce on top of the cooked pasta.

Per Serving:
calories: 181 | fat: 1g | protein: 9g | carbs: 40g | fiber: 7g

Baked Tempeh Nuggets

Prep time: 15 minutes | **Cook time:** 30 minutes | Serves 4

- 1 (8-ounce / 227-g) package tempeh, lightly steamed if desired
- ¼ cup almond milk
- ¼ cup nutritional yeast
- 1 tablespoon Fall & Winter All-Purpose Seasoning or other seasoning blend
- 1 teaspoon arrowroot powder
- 1 teaspoon fresh lemon juice
- ¼ teaspoon black pepper
- ¼ teaspoon hot sauce
- ¼ teaspoon salt (optional)
- 1 cup whole wheat bread crumbs

1. Preheat the oven to 400°F (205°C). Prepare a baking sheet by lining it with parchment paper. 2. Cut the tempeh in half and then quarter each half to create 8 pieces. Gently press down on each piece with your hand to flatten them slightly, increasing the surface area and giving them a nugget-like shape. 3. In a shallow dish, combine almond milk, nutritional yeast, seasoning blend, arrowroot powder, lemon juice, pepper, hot sauce, and salt (if desired). Add the tempeh nuggets to the mixture and let them soak for 5 minutes, ensuring each piece is well coated by turning them over. 4. Place bread crumbs in another shallow dish. Using one hand for the wet ingredients and the other for the dry, transfer each piece of tempeh from the batter to the bread crumbs. Then, place them on the prepared baking sheet. 5. Bake for 30 minutes, flipping the nuggets halfway through, until they turn golden brown on both sides. Serve.

Per Serving:
calories: 267 | fat: 8g | protein: 19g | carbs: 32g | fiber: 3g

Fried Rice with Tofu Scramble

Prep time: 15 minutes | **Cook time:** 35 minutes | Serves 2

- 4 cups cooked quick-cooking brown rice
- 1 cup cooked or canned green peas
- 1 (7-ounce / 198-g) pack extra-firm tofu, scrambled
- 1 cup julienned carrots
- ¼ cup curry spices
- 1 cup water
- Optional Toppings:
- Lemon slices
- Sauerkraut
- Fresh cilantro

1. Cook 1½ cups of brown rice for approximately 25 minutes. 2. Heat a large nonstick frying pan over medium heat and add ½ cup of water along with the tofu scramble. 3. Sprinkle in the curry spices and cook for about 5 minutes, stirring occasionally to prevent the tofu from sticking to the pan. Continue cooking until the tofu is thoroughly heated and most of the water has evaporated. 4. Add the carrots, rice, and green peas to the pan, along with the remaining ½ cup of water. Stir-fry for another 5 minutes or until the water has evaporated. 5. Turn off the heat, divide the fried rice evenly between 2 bowls, and serve with optional toppings. Enjoy! 6. If there are any leftovers, store the fried rice in an airtight container in the refrigerator and consume within 3 days. Alternatively, you can store it in the freezer for up to 30 days. Thaw the frozen fried rice at room temperature before reheating it in a nonstick frying pan or using a microwave.

Per Serving:
calories: 286 | fat: 10g | protein: 18g | carbs: 30g | fiber: 8g

Barley and White Bean Pilaf

Prep time: 15 minutes | **Cook time:** 55 minutes | Serves 4

- 1 medium yellow onion, peeled and finely diced
- 1 celery stalk, finely diced
- 1 medium carrot, peeled and finely diced
- 1½ cups pearled barley
- 2-inch piece orange peel
- 1 cinnamon stick
- 3 cups vegetable stock, or low-sodium vegetable broth
- 2 cups cooked navy or other white beans, or 1 (15-ounce / 425-g) can, drained and rinsed
- ¼ cup finely chopped dill

1. Place the onion, celery, and carrot in a large saucepan and sauté over medium heat for 7 to 8 minutes. Add water 1 to 2 tablespoons at a time to keep the vegetables from sticking to the pan. Add the barley, orange peel, cinnamon stick, and vegetable stock and bring the pan to a boil over high heat. 2. Reduce the heat to medium and cook for 35 minutes. Add the beans and cook for another 10 minutes, until the barley is tender. Remove from the heat and stir in the dill.

Per Serving:
calories: 418 | fat: 1g | protein: 15g | carbs: 78g | fiber: 18g

Red Lentil Dal

Prep time: 15 minutes | **Cook time:** 35 minutes | Serves 4

- 1 large yellow onion, peeled and diced
- 2 cloves garlic, peeled and minced
- 1 bay leaf
- 1 tablespoon grated ginger
- 1 teaspoon turmeric
- 1 tablespoon cumin seeds, toasted and ground
- 1 tablespoon coriander seeds, toasted and ground
- ½ teaspoon crushed red pepper flakes
- 2 cup red lentils, rinsed
- Salt, to taste (optional)
- Zest of 1 lemon

1. In a large saucepan, sauté the onion over medium heat for 10 minutes. To prevent sticking, add water 1 to 2 tablespoons at a time. Afterward, add the garlic, bay leaf, ginger, turmeric, cumin, coriander, and crushed red pepper flakes. Cook for an additional minute. 2. Add the lentils and 4 cups of water to the pot. Bring it to a boil over high heat. Then, reduce the heat to medium and cover the pot. Allow it to cook for 20 to 25 minutes, or until the lentils are tender and starting to break down. Remove from heat. If desired, season with salt and add lemon zest.

Per Serving:
calories: 379 | fat: 2g | protein: 24g | carbs: 68g | fiber: 12g

North African Chickpeas and Vegetables

Prep time: 35 minutes | Cook time: 25 minutes | Serves 4

Chermoula Sauce:
1 large tomato, chopped
½ cup Kalamata olives, pitted
1 cup chopped cilantro
6 cloves garlic, peeled and minced
Zest of 1 lemon and juice of 2 lemons
1 tablespoon sweet paprika
2 teaspoons ground coriander
2 teaspoons ground cumin
¼ teaspoon cayenne pepper, or to taste
Salt, to taste (optional)
Vegetables:
1 medium yellow onion, peeled and cut into ½-inch rings
1 medium red bell pepper, seeded and cut into ½-inch strips
8 ounces (227 g) button mushrooms, sliced
1 medium zucchini, halved lengthwise and cut into ½-inch slices
1 medium yellow squash, halved lengthwise and cut into ½-inch slices
2 cups cooked chickpeas, or 1 (15-ounce / 425-g) can, drained and rinsed
Salt and freshly ground black pepper, to taste

Make the Chermoula Sauce:
1. In a blender, combine tomato, olives, cilantro, garlic, lemon zest and juice, paprika, coriander, cumin, cayenne pepper, and salt (if desired). Process the ingredients until smooth and creamy. Set the sauce aside.

Make the Vegetables:
2. Heat a large saucepan over medium-high heat. Add onion, red pepper, and mushrooms to the pan and sauté them for 8 to 10 minutes. To prevent sticking, add water 1 to 2 tablespoons at a time. 3. Add zucchini, yellow squash, and chickpeas to the pan and cook for an additional 10 minutes. 4. Stir in the chermoula sauce and continue cooking for another 5 minutes. 5. Season with salt and pepper to taste.

Per Serving:
calories: 212 | fat: 5g | protein: 11g | carbs: 34g | fiber: 9g

Chana Saag

Prep time: 20 minutes | Cook time: 30 minutes | Serves 4

1 medium yellow onion, peeled and diced small
1 jalapeño pepper, minced (for less heat, remove the seeds)
3 cloves garlic, peeled and minced
1 tablespoon grated ginger
2 teaspoons ground cumin
1 teaspoon ground coriander
1 teaspoon turmeric
1 teaspoon fenugreek
1 teaspoon crushed red pepper flakes, or to taste
1 large tomato, finely chopped
1 cup unsweetened plain almond milk
2 pounds (907 g) fresh spinach, chopped (about 12 cups)
2 cups cooked chickpeas, or 1 (15-ounce / 425-g) can, drained and rinsed
Salt, to taste (optional)

1. In a large saucepan, place the onion and sauté over medium-high heat for 8 to 10 minutes until it becomes browned. To prevent sticking, add water 1 to 2 tablespoons at a time. 2. Reduce the heat to medium-low and add the jalapeño pepper, garlic, ginger, cumin, coriander, turmeric, fenugreek, and crushed red pepper flakes. Stir frequently and cook for 4 minutes, adding water only as needed. 3. Add the tomato to the pan and cook for another 5 minutes. Then, add almond milk, spinach, and chickpeas. Cover the pot and reduce the heat to medium-low. Cook for approximately 10 minutes or until the spinach is wilted. If desired, season with salt.

Per Serving:
calories: 235 | fat: 3g | protein: 16g | carbs: 39g | fiber: 12g

Mixed Beans Chili

Prep time: 20 minutes | Cook time: 1 hour | Serves 6

1 pound (454 g) beans, mixed varieties
1 tablespoon extra virgin olive oil (optional)
½ cup diced onion
4 cloves garlic, finely chopped
4 cups vegetable broth, more if needed
1 (28 ounces / 794 g) can crushed fire-roasted tomatoes
1 (8 ounces / 227 g) can tomato sauce
1 (6 ounces / 170 g) can tomato paste
2 tablespoons vegan Worcestershire sauce
2 tablespoons chili powder
2 teaspoons ground cumin
1½ teaspoons dried oregano
¼ teaspoon ground cloves
½ teaspoon cayenne pepper
1 teaspoon salt (optional)

1. Rinse the beans and place them in a large stockpot. Add enough water to cover the beans by about 3 inches. Allow the beans to soak overnight, as they will expand.
2. Drain the soaked beans and return them to the stockpot. 3. If desired, heat oil in a large skillet over medium-high heat. Add the onion and sauté until translucent, which should take around 10 to 15 minutes. Add the garlic and sauté for an additional minute. Transfer this mixture to the stockpot with the beans. Add vegetable broth, crushed tomatoes, tomato sauce, tomato paste, and Worcestershire sauce. The liquid should cover the beans by a couple of inches. If needed, you can add more broth or water. Stir well to combine. Add the remaining ingredients and stir again. Cover the pot and bring it to a boil. 4. Once boiling, remove the lid, reduce the heat to low, and simmer gently. The heat should be so low that the liquid barely moves. Do not cover the pot again, as it will enhance the flavor. If the liquid reduces and the beans are no longer submerged, add more broth or water. However, if you add more liquid, cover the pot again, raise the heat to bring it to a boil, then immediately reduce the heat and uncover. Make sure the heat is not too high. Cook for 45 minutes and check the tenderness of the beans. They should be tender. If they are not done yet, continue cooking for a longer period of time, but it shouldn't exceed 1 hour.

Per Serving:
calories: 117 | fat: 4g | protein: 20g | carbs: 21g | fiber: 7g

Mujadara (Lentils with Rice and Caramelized Onions)

Prep time: 10 minutes | Cook time: 2 hours | Serves 4

- 1½ cups green lentils, rinsed
- ¾ teaspoon ground cinnamon
- ½ teaspoon ground allspice
- ¾ cup brown basmati rice
- 3 large yellow onions, peeled and diced
- Salt and freshly ground black pepper, to taste

1. In a large pot, combine lentils and 5 cups of water. Bring it to a boil over high heat, then reduce the heat to medium and let it simmer for 30 minutes. Add cinnamon and allspice, and continue cooking for another 15 to 20 minutes until the lentils are tender. 2. In a separate medium saucepan, bring 1½ cups of water to a boil. Add rice to the boiling water and bring it back to a boil over high heat. Reduce the heat to medium and cook the rice, covered, for approximately 45 minutes or until it becomes tender. 3. Heat a large skillet over high heat. Add onions to the skillet and cook, stirring frequently, for about 10 minutes. To prevent sticking, add water 1 to 2 tablespoons at a time. Reduce the heat to medium-low and continue cooking until the onions are browned, which should take around 10 minutes. Add the cooked lentils and rice to the skillet with the onions and mix everything well. Season with salt and pepper to taste.

Per Serving:
calories: 405 | fat: 1g | protein: 21g | carbs: 77g | fiber: 10g

Fancy Rice

Prep time: 10 minutes | Cook time: 40 minutes | Serves 4

- 1 cup uncooked wild and brown rice blend, rinsed
- 2 teaspoons virgin olive oil (optional)
- 1 teaspoon apple cider vinegar
- ½ teaspoon ground coriander
- ¼ teaspoon ground sumac
- ¼ cup unsweetened dried cranberries
- ¼ cup chopped fresh flat-leaf parsley
- 2 green onions, thinly sliced
- Salt and pepper, to taste (optional)
- ¼ cup almonds, chopped, for garnish

1. In a medium saucepan, place the wild and brown rice blend. Add enough cold water to cover the rice by 1 inch. Bring it to a boil, then reduce the heat to a simmer and cover the saucepan. Cook the rice for approximately 40 minutes or until all the liquid is absorbed. Once cooked, remove the saucepan from the heat and let the rice sit for 5 minutes. Fluff the rice with a fork and transfer it gently to a medium bowl. 2. To the cooked rice, add olive oil, apple cider vinegar, coriander, sumac, dried cranberries, parsley, green onions, and salt and pepper (if desired). Toss the ingredients gently to combine. Garnish the rice with chopped almonds. Serve the rice warm.

Per Serving:
calories: 252 | fat: 7g | protein: 5g | carbs: 25g | fiber: 3g

Bulgur Chickpea Pilaf

Prep time: 15 minutes | Cook time: 35 minutes | Serves 4

- 1 medium yellow onion, peeled and diced small
- 3 cloves garlic, peeled and minced
- 1½ tablespoons grated ginger
- 1½ cups bulgur
- 3 cups vegetable stock, or low-sodium vegetable broth
- 2 cups cooked chickpeas, or 1 (15-ounce / 425-g) can, drained and rinsed
- 1 Roma tomato, chopped
- Zest and juice of 1 lemon
- Salt and freshly ground black pepper, to taste
- 4 green onions (white and green parts), thinly sliced

1. Place the onion in a large saucepan and sauté over medium heat for 10 minutes. Add water 1 to 2 tablespoons at a time to keep the onion from sticking to the pan. Stir in the garlic and ginger and cook for 30 seconds. Add the bulgur and vegetable stock and bring to a boil over high heat. Reduce the heat to medium and cook, covered, until the bulgur is tender, about 15 minutes. 2. Stir in the chickpeas, tomato, and lemon zest and juice and cook for another 5 minutes. Season with salt and pepper and serve garnished with the green onions.

Per Serving:
calories: 344 | fat: 2g | protein: 14g | carbs: 69g | fiber: 13g

Mac 'N' Mince

Prep time: 15 minutes | Cook time: 10 minutes | Serves 4

- 2 cups whole wheat macaroni
- 1 (7-ounce / 198-g) pack textured soy mince
- ½ cup tahini
- ¼ cup nutritional yeast
- 2 tablespoons lemon garlic pepper seasoning
- ½ cup water
- 2 tablespoons turmeric (optional)
- Optional Toppings:
- Sun-dried tomatoes
- Crispy onions

1. Cook the macaroni and set it aside afterwards. 2. Put a nonstick deep frying pan over medium high heat and add the soy mince with the ¼ cup of water. 3. Stir fry the soy mince until it is cooked and most of the water has evaporated. 4. Add the tahini, ¼ cup of water, nutritional yeast, lemon garlic pepper seasoning and the optional turmeric to the soy mince. 5. Cook a little longer, stirring continuously, until everything is well combined. 6. Add the cooked macaroni to the pan with soy mince and stir thoroughly until the mac 'N' mince is mixed well. 7. Divide the mac 'N' mince between two plates, serve with the optional toppings and enjoy! 8. Store the mac 'N' mince in an airtight container in the fridge, and consume within 3 days. Alternatively, store it in the freezer for a maximum of 30 days and thaw at room temperature. Use a microwave, toaster oven, or frying pan to reheat the mac 'n' mince.

Per Serving:
calories: 454 | fat: 20g | protein: 25g | carbs: 42g | fiber: 10g

Mexican Quinoa Bowl

Prep time: 10 minutes | Cook time: 22 minutes | Serves 2

1 cup cooked or canned chickpeas
1 cup cooked or canned black beans
½ cup dry quinoa
2 cups vegetable stock
2 tablespoons Mexican chorizo seasoning
Optional Toppings:
lime juice
fresh cilantro
avocado slices

1. When using dry chickpeas and beans, soak and cook ⅓ cup of dry chickpeas and black beans. 2. Put a large pot over medium-high heat and add the vegetable stock to the pot along with the quinoa. 3. Bring to a boil, then turn the heat down to medium. 4. Cook the quinoa for about 15 minutes, without covering the pot, and stir occasionally. 5. Add the Mexican chorizo seasoning, black beans and chickpeas, and cook for another 7 minutes, stirring occasionally. 6. Turn the heat off and let it cool down for a minute. 7. Divide between 2 bowls, garnish with the optional toppings, serve and enjoy! 8. Store in an airtight container in the fridge, and consume within 2 days. Alternatively, store in the freezer for a maximum of 30 days and thaw at room temperature. The bowl can be served cold or reheated in a saucepan or a microwave.

Per Serving:
calories: 487 | fat: 8g | protein: 23g | carbs: 80g | fiber: 19g

Kasha Varnishkes (Buckwheat Groats with Bow-Tie Pasta)

Prep time: 20 minutes | Cook time: 35 minutes | Serves 4

2 cups vegetable stock, or low-sodium vegetable broth
1 cup buckwheat groats
1 large yellow onion, peeled and diced small
8 ounces (227 g) button mushrooms, sliced
½ pound (227 g) whole-grain farfalle, cooked according to package directions, drained, and kept warm
2 tablespoons finely chopped dill
Salt and freshly ground black pepper, to taste

1. Place the vegetable stock in a medium saucepan and bring to a boil over high heat. Add the buckwheat groats and bring the pot back to a boil over high heat. Reduce the heat to medium and cook, uncovered, until the groats are tender, about 12 to 15 minutes. 2. Place the onion in a large saucepan and sauté over medium heat until well browned, about 15 minutes. Add water 1 to 2 tablespoons at a time to keep the onion from sticking, but use as little water as possible. Add the mushrooms and cook for another 5 minutes. Remove from the heat. Add the cooked pasta, buckwheat groats, and dill. Season with salt and pepper.

Per Serving:
calories: 240 | fat: 1g | protein: 8g | carbs: 51g | fiber: 6g

Farro Tabbouleh

Prep time: 15 minutes | Cook time: 30 minutes | Serves 6

2½ cups water or vegetable broth
1 cup farro, soaked overnight and drained
3 scallions, sliced thin
1 English cucumber, diced
1 red or yellow bell pepper, finely diced
1 bunch flat-leaf parsley leaves, chopped
Handful mint leaves, chopped
Grated zest and juice of 2 lemons
¼ cup vegetable broth
¼ teaspoon salt (optional)
⅛ teaspoon black pepper

1. In a medium saucepan, combine water and farro. Bring it to a boil and then reduce the heat to low. Cover the saucepan and cook the farro, stirring occasionally, until it reaches an al dente texture, which usually takes about 25 minutes. 2. Let the cooked farro cool for 10 minutes, then transfer it to a large bowl. Add the remaining ingredients to the bowl and toss everything together to combine. Serve immediately. Please note that if you refrigerate the tabbouleh, the herbs may discolor. It can be stored in the refrigerator for up to 2 days.

Per Serving:
calories: 115 | fat: 1g | protein: 4g | carbs: 26g | fiber: 5g

Hearty Veggie Hoagies

Prep time: 10 minutes | Cook time: 5 minutes | Makes 1 baguette

1 (12-ounce / 340-g) sourdough or whole grain baguette
2 sliced tomatoes
1 cucumber, sliced, salted, and drained
1 cup canned or frozen and thawed artichoke hearts, roughly chopped
1 red bell pepper, sliced into rings
¼ small red onion, thinly sliced
⅓ cup Kalamata olives, pitted and chopped
Salt and black pepper (optional)
2 tablespoons pesto
Balsamic vinegar

1. Slice the baguette in half horizontally, then slice off the top third from each half. Scoop out some of the insides of the bottom portion, reserving them for another use (such as bread crumbs). 2. Toast lightly. 3. Meanwhile, combine the tomatoes, cucumber, artichokes, bell pepper, onion, and olives in a medium bowl and season with salt (if desired) and pepper to taste. 4. Spread the vegetables inside the bottom section of the baguette (being mindful not to add too much liquid). 5. Spread the pesto on the cut side of the baguette top. Drizzle the contents of the bottom with a bit of balsamic, then place the baguette top onto the vegetables. 6. Wrap tightly in parchment paper, then aluminum foil. For best flavor, let sit for at least 1 hour or up to 12 hours. Slice and serve.

Per Serving: (¼ baguette)
calories: 331 | fat: 8g | protein: 12g | carbs: 55g | fiber: 5g

Spiced Kidney Bean Curry

Prep time: 5 minutes | **Cook time:** 20 minutes | **Serves 4**

- 1 teaspoon extra-virgin olive oil (optional)
- 2 garlic cloves, minced
- 2 teaspoons minced fresh ginger
- 1 small yellow onion, chopped small
- 2 (15-ounce / 425-g) cans kidney beans, drained and rinsed
- 3 teaspoons curry powder
- ½ teaspoon salt (optional)
- 1 (15-ounce / 425-g) can crushed tomatoes
- 2 cups water
- 4 generous tablespoons chopped fresh cilantro, for garnish
- Red pepper flakes, for garnish (optional)

1. In a large saucepan or wok, heat the olive oil over medium heat. Add the garlic, ginger, and onion and cook until the onions are browned, about 7 minutes. Add the kidney beans, curry powder, salt (if using), tomatoes, and water, raise the heat to high, and bring to a boil, stirring often. 2. Turn the heat to low and, using a potato masher, gently mash the ingredients to break up some of the beans, which will help thicken the curry, and simmer for 10 minutes. Spoon the curry into bowls, garnish with cilantro and red pepper flakes (if using), and serve.

Per Serving:
calories: 230 | fat: 2g | protein: 14g | carbs: 42g | fiber: 12g

Eggplant and Chickpea Rice Pilaf

Prep time: 20 minutes | **Cook time:** 1 hour 10 minutes | **Serves 4**

- 2 cups vegetable stock, or low-sodium vegetable broth
- 1 cup brown basmati rice
- 1 large yellow onion, peeled and diced small
- 6 cloves garlic, peeled and minced
- 2 jalapeño peppers, seeded and minced
- 1 tablespoon cumin seeds, toasted and ground
- 1 tablespoon ground coriander
- 1 teaspoon turmeric
- 1 large eggplant, stemmed and cut into ½-inch cubes
- 2 cups cooked chickpeas, or 1 (15-ounce / 425-g) can, drained and rinsed
- ¼ cup finely chopped mint
- ½ cup finely chopped basil
- Salt, to taste (optional)
- ½ cup finely chopped cilantro

1. Bring the vegetable stock to a boil in a medium saucepan. Add the rice and bring the mixture back to a boil over high heat. Reduce the heat to medium and cook, covered, until the rice is tender, about 45 minutes. 2. Place the onion in a large saucepan and sauté over medium heat for 7 to 8 minutes. Add water 1 to 2 tablespoons at a time to keep the onion from sticking to the pan. Add the garlic, jalapeño peppers, cumin, coriander, turmeric, and eggplant and cook until the eggplant is tender, about 12 minutes. Add the cooked rice, chickpeas, mint, and basil. Season with salt (if using) and serve garnished with the cilantro.

Per Serving:
calories: 373 | fat: 4g | protein: 13g | carbs: 73g | fiber: 12g

Pasta Marinara with Spicy Italian Bean Balls

Prep time: 20 minutes | **Cook time:** 35 minutes | **Serves 4**

Spicy Italian Bean Balls:
- ¼ cup vegetable broth
- ½ yellow onion, minced
- 2 teaspoons dried oregano
- 1 teaspoon fennel seeds
- 1 teaspoon garlic powder
- ½ teaspoon crushed red pepper
- 1 (15-ounce / 425-g) can white beans, drained and rinsed
- Salt and black pepper (optional)
- ½ cup whole-grain bread crumbs

Weeknight Marinara:
- 2 tablespoons mushroom stock
- Handful basil leaves
- 3 garlic cloves, minced
- 1 (28-ounce / 794-g) can whole tomatoes with juice reserved
- Salt (optional)
- Pasta

1. To make the bean balls, preheat the oven to 350ºF (180ºC). Line a baking sheet with parchment paper. 2. Heat a medium skillet over medium heat, then add the broth. Add the onion and cook, stirring often, until it begins to soften, about 5 minutes. 3. Add the oregano, fennel seeds, garlic powder, and crushed red pepper. Cook until fragrant, about 1 minute longer. Remove from the heat and transfer to a food processor along with the beans. 4. Pulse to combine and season with salt (if desired) and pepper to taste; add the bread crumbs. Pulse until just combined. 5. Using a 2-ounce (57-g) cookie scoop, form balls (it may be necessary to wet hands to prevent sticking). Bake for 15 minutes, flip, and bake 15 minutes longer, or until golden brown. 6. Meanwhile, make the marinara: Place a medium saucepan over medium-high heat. Add the stock to the hot pan. Once it's warm, add the basil and garlic and cook for 2 minutes, stirring occasionally. Stir in the tomatoes with their juice, bring just to a boil, then reduce heat to low, cover, and cook for 15 minutes. Season with salt, if desired. 7. Cook the pasta according to package instructions. Serve topped with the bean balls.

Per Serving:
calories: 311 | fat: 3g | protein: 16g | carbs: 58g | fiber: 12g

Southwest Stuffed Peppers

Prep time: 10 minutes | **Cook time:** 30 minutes | **Serves 4**

- 4 bell peppers
- 3 cups cooked brown rice
- 1 cup cooked black beans
- 1 cup fresh or frozen corn
- 1 cup vegetable broth
- 2 tablespoons tomato paste
- 2 tablespoons chili powder
- 1 teaspoon ground cumin

1. Preheat the oven to 375ºF (190ºC). 2. Cut the tops off the bell peppers, and remove any seeds or fibers that remain inside the core or inside the tops of the peppers. 3. In a large bowl, mix together the rice, beans, corn, broth, tomato paste, chili powder, and cumin until the tomato paste and spices have been thoroughly incorporated. 4. Spoon one-quarter of the rice mixture into each pepper. Set the peppers upright on a baking dish, and place the tops back onto the peppers. 5. Bake for 1 hour, or until the peppers are easily pierced with a fork, and serve.

Per Serving:
calories: 270 | fat: 3g | protein: 11g | carbs: 55g | fiber: 9g

Chapter 5
Desserts

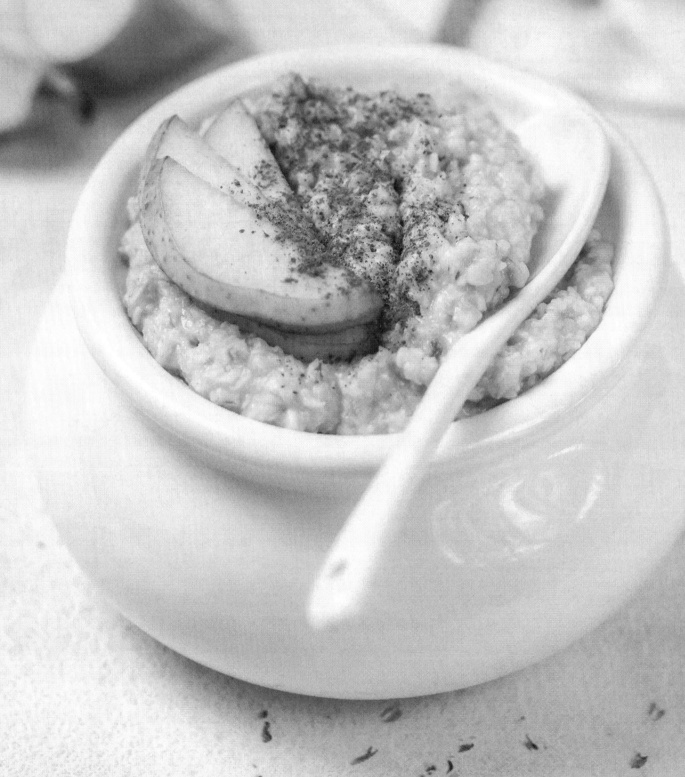

Vanilla Bean Whip

Prep time: 5 minutes | Cook time: 0 minutes | Makes 2 cups

1 (12-ounce / 340-g) package extra-firm silken tofu, drained
½ cup cashews, soaked overnight and drained
½ cup 100% pure maple syrup (optional)
2 tablespoons fresh lemon juice
Pinch salt (optional)
1 vanilla bean

1. In a blender, combine tofu, cashews, maple syrup (if desired), lemon juice, and salt (if desired). Blend until the mixture becomes smooth. Make sure to scrape down the sides of the blender to incorporate all the ingredients. 2. Using a sharp knife, slice the vanilla bean in half lengthwise and scrape out the seeds. Add the vanilla seeds to the blender and blend the mixture again until it becomes very smooth. 3. Transfer the mixture from the blender to a bowl and cover it with plastic wrap. Place the bowl in the refrigerator and let it chill for several hours, or until it becomes firm.

Per Serving:
calories: 143 | fat: 6g | protein: 5g | carbs: 17g | fiber: 0g

Almond Anise Biscotti

Prep time: 5 minutes | Cook time: 40 minutes | Makes 18 slices

⅓ cup unsweetened plant-based milk
2 tablespoons ground flaxseeds
¾ cup date sugar (optional)
¼ cup unsweetened applesauce
¼ cup almond butter
½ teaspoon pure vanilla extract
½ teaspoon almond extract
1⅔ cups whole wheat pastry flour
2 tablespoons cornstarch
2 teaspoons baking powder
2 teaspoons anise seeds
½ teaspoon salt (optional)
1 cup slivered almonds

1. Preheat your oven to 350ºF (180ºC) and line a baking sheet with parchment paper or a Silpat baking mat. 2. In a large mixing bowl, vigorously mix together the plant-based milk and flaxseeds using a fork until frothy. Add in the date sugar (if desired), applesauce, almond butter, vanilla, and almond extract. Mix well. 3. Sift in the flour, cornstarch, and baking powder. Add the anise seeds and salt (if desired). Mix everything together until well combined. Knead in the almonds using your hands as the dough will be stiff. 4. On the prepared baking sheet, shape the dough into a rectangle measuring about 12 inches long and 3 to 4 inches wide. Bake for 26 to 28 minutes, or until lightly puffed and browned. Remove from the oven and let it cool on the baking sheet for 30 minutes. 5. Increase the oven temperature to 375ºF (190ºC). Using a heavy and sharp knife, slice the biscotti loaf into ½-inch-thick slices. It's best to do this in one motion by pushing down instead of sawing to prevent crumbling. Place the slices back on the baking sheet and bake for 10 to 12 minutes, flipping them halfway through. Allow the slices to cool for a few minutes on the baking sheet before transferring them to cooling racks.

Per Serving:
calories: 127 | fat: 5g | protein: 3g | carbs: 16g | fiber: 2g

Better-Than-Mom's Banana Bread

Prep time: 5 minutes | Cook time: 1 hour | Makes one 8 × 4-inch loaf

2 cups whole wheat pastry flour
¾ teaspoon baking soda
¾ teaspoon salt (optional)
1 cup mashed banana
½ cup 100% pure maple syrup (optional)
⅓ cup unsweetened applesauce
¼ cup unsweetened plant-based milk
1½ teaspoons pure vanilla extract

1. Preheat the oven to 350ºF (180ºC). Have ready an 8 × 4-inch nonstick or silicone baking pan. 2. In a large mixing bowl, sift together the flour, baking soda, and salt (if using). 3. In a separate mixing bowl, combine the mashed banana, maple syrup (if using), applesauce, plant-based milk, and vanilla. 4. Make a well in the center of the dry ingredients and pour in the wet ingredients, mixing just until everything is evenly moistened. 5. Spoon the batter into the prepared loaf pan. Distribute the batter evenly along the length of the pan but don't spread the batter to the edges; the batter will spread as it bakes. Bake for 55 to 60 minutes. It's hard to test for doneness with a knife because the banana tends to stay moist, so judge by the edges of bread. They should be golden brown and pulling away from the sides of the pan. 6. Let the bread cool for at least 30 minutes, then run a knife around the edges and carefully invert the loaf onto a cooling rack. Be sure it is fully cooled before slicing.

Per Serving:
calories: 125 | fat: 0g | protein: 3g | carbs: 23g | fiber: 2g

Almond-Date Energy Bites

Prep time: 5 minutes | Cook time: 0 minutes | Makes 24 bites

1 cup dates, pitted
1 cup unsweetened shredded coconut
¼ cup chia seeds
¾ cup ground almonds
¼ cup cocoa nibs or nondairy chocolate chips

1. In a food processor, blend all the ingredients until they become crumbly and stick together. Make sure to push down the sides of the processor as needed to ensure even blending. If you don't have a food processor, you can mash soft Medjool dates by hand. However, if you're using harder baking dates, you may need to soak them first and then attempt to purée them in a blender. 2. Take the mixture and shape it into 24 balls. Place the balls on a baking sheet lined with parchment or waxed paper. Refrigerate the balls for approximately 15 minutes to allow them to set.

Per Serving: (1 bite)
calories: 53 | fat: 3g | protein: 0g | carbs: 6g | fiber: 1g

Banana Soft Serve

Prep time: 5 minutes | **Cook time:** 0 minutes | **Serves 2**

2 ripe bananas, peeled, sliced, and frozen
Optional Toppings:
Drizzle of nondairy chocolate sauce
1 handful chopped unsalted roasted peanuts

1. Using a food processor or high-powered blender, pulse or blend the frozen sliced bananas until they reach a thick and creamy consistency, resembling ice cream.
2. Scoop the banana "ice cream" into a bowl or ice cream cone. Feel free to add your favorite toppings such as chocolate chips, nuts, or fruit. Enjoy your delicious treat immediately.

Per Serving:
calories: 105 | fat: 0g | protein: 1g | carbs: 27g | fiber: 3g

Caramel-Coconut Frosted Brownies

Prep time: 10 minutes | **Cook time:** 25 minutes | **Makes 12 brownies**

Brownies:
1 (15-ounce / 425-g) can black beans, drained and rinsed
½ cup rolled oats
6 tablespoons pure maple syrup
⅓ cup cocoa powder
⅓ cup unsweetened applesauce
2 tablespoons unsalted, unsweetened almond butter
1 teaspoon vanilla extract
Pinch ground cinnamon
Frosting:
1 cup pitted dates
6 tablespoons unsweetened plant-based milk
2 tablespoons nutritional yeast
¼ teaspoon vanilla extract
⅛ teaspoon red miso paste
¼ cup chopped pecans
3 tablespoons unsweetened coconut flakes

Make the Brownies:
1. Preheat your oven to 350°F (180°C) and line a 12-cup cupcake tin with liners.
2. In a food processor, combine the beans, oats, maple syrup, cocoa powder, applesauce, almond butter, vanilla, and cinnamon. Process the mixture until it becomes smooth. 3. Transfer the mixture to the prepared cupcake tin, starting with about 2 tablespoons per cup, and then evenly divide the remaining mixture among the cups. 4. Bake the brownies for 20 to 22 minutes, or until the tops become crispy and a toothpick inserted into the center of a cupcake comes out mostly clean. Once baked, remove the brownies from the tin and transfer them to a wire rack. Let them cool for approximately 5 minutes.
Make the Frosting:
5. While the brownies are cooling, in a food processor, combine the dates, milk, nutritional yeast, vanilla, and miso. Process the mixture until it becomes mostly smooth. 6. Pulse in the pecans and coconut until well mixed, but with some texture remaining. 7. Spread approximately 1 heaping tablespoon of the frosting onto each brownie. Serve and enjoy!

Per Serving:
calories: 235 | fat: 11g | protein: 10g | carbs: 30g | fiber: 12g

Pumpkin Bread Pudding

Prep time: 10 minutes | **Cook time:** 25 minutes | **Serves 8**

1¼ cups pumpkin purée (a little over ½ of a 15-ounce / 425-g can)
1 cup unsweetened plant-based milk
½ cup 100% maple syrup (optional)
2 teaspoons pure vanilla extract
2 tablespoons cornstarch
½ teaspoon salt (optional)
½ teaspoon ground cinnamon
¾ teaspoon ground ginger
¼ teaspoon ground nutmeg
¼ teaspoon ground allspice
⅛ teaspoon ground cloves
8 slices stale whole wheat bread, cut into 1-inch cubes (about 6 cups)
½ cup golden raisins

1. Preheat the oven to 350°F (180°C) and prepare an 8 × 8-inch nonstick or silicone baking pan. 2. In a large bowl, whisk together pumpkin puree, plant-based milk, maple syrup (if using), and vanilla. Add cornstarch, salt (if using), cinnamon, ginger, nutmeg, allspice, and cloves. Whisk everything together until well combined. Stir in bread cubes and raisins, ensuring they are coated evenly. 3. Transfer the mixture to the prepared pan and bake for approximately 25 minutes, or until the top turns golden brown and feels firm to the touch. Serve the dish while warm.

Per Serving:
calories: 192 | fat: 1g | protein: 4g | carbs: 31g | fiber: 2g

Zesty Orange-Cranberry Energy Bites

Prep time: 10 minutes | **Cook time:** 0 minutes | **Makes 12 bites**

2 tablespoons almond butter, or cashew or sunflower seed butter
2 tablespoons maple syrup or brown rice syrup (optional)
¾ cup cooked quinoa
¼ cup sesame seeds, toasted
1 tablespoon chia seeds
½ teaspoon almond extract or vanilla extract
Zest of 1 orange
1 tablespoon dried cranberries
¼ cup ground almonds

1. In a medium bowl, combine the nut or seed butter with syrup (if desired) and mix until you achieve a smooth and creamy consistency. 2. Add the remaining ingredients to the bowl and stir well to ensure that the mixture holds together as a ball. 3. Shape the mixture into 12 balls and place them on a baking sheet lined with parchment or waxed paper. Refrigerate the balls for approximately 15 minutes to allow them to set.

Per Serving: (1 bite)
calories: 71 | fat: 4g | protein: 2g | carbs: 6g | fiber: 1g

Cherry Chocolate Bark

Prep time: 5 minutes | Cook time: 0 minutes | Serves 8

- 1 cup vegan semisweet chocolate chips
- 1 cup sliced almonds
- 1 cup dried tart cherries, chopped
- ½ teaspoon flaky sea salt, for sprinkling (optional)

1. Prepare a rimmed baking sheet by lining it with parchment paper and place it in the fridge or freezer to become very cold. 2. In a heatproof glass bowl, set it over a pan of simmering water to create a double boiler. Add the chocolate to the bowl and melt it slowly, stirring occasionally. Be cautious not to let any water droplets enter the bowl, as it may cause the chocolate to seize. 3. Once some pieces of unmelted chocolate still remain, remove the bowl from the heat source (or microwave). Stir the chocolate well until the remaining pieces melt, but avoid stirring too vigorously to prevent the formation of air bubbles. 4. Pour the melted chocolate onto the chilled prepared pan and use a thin spatula to spread it evenly, leaving a small border around the edges. Sprinkle the almonds and cherries evenly over the chocolate, followed by a sprinkle of salt if desired. Place the pan in the refrigerator until the chocolate becomes firm. 5. Break the chocolate bark into pieces and store them in an airtight container in the refrigerator for up to 1 week.

Per Serving:
calories: 189 | fat: 12g | protein: 3g | carbs: 17g | fiber: 3g

Pumpkin Spice Bread

Prep time: 5 minutes | Cook time: 1 hour | Makes one 8 × 4-inch loaf

- 2 cups whole wheat pastry flour
- 2 teaspoons baking powder
- 1 teaspoon baking soda
- 2 teaspoons ground cinnamon
- ½ teaspoon ground ginger
- ¼ teaspoon ground allspice
- ⅛ teaspoon ground cloves
- ½ cup chopped walnuts (optional)
- 1 (15-ounce / 425-g) can pumpkin purée (about 2 cups)
- ½ cup 100% pure maple syrup (optional)
- ⅓ cup apple butter
- 1 teaspoon pure vanilla extract
- ½ cup golden raisins (optional)

1. Preheat your oven to 350°F (180°C) and prepare an 8 × 4-inch nonstick or silicone baking pan. 2. In a large mixing bowl, sift together the flour, baking powder, baking soda, cinnamon, ginger, allspice, and cloves. 3. In a separate mixing bowl, vigorously mix together the pumpkin, maple syrup (if desired), apple butter, and vanilla. 4. Pour the wet mixture into the dry mixture and combine until all the ingredients are evenly moistened. The batter will be stiff. If using, fold in the raisins and walnuts. 5. Spoon the batter into the prepared loaf pan, making sure to distribute it evenly along the length of the pan without spreading it to the edges. The batter will spread as it bakes. Bake for 50 to 60 minutes, or until a knife inserted into the center comes out clean. 6. Remove the pan from the oven and allow the bread to cool for at least 30 minutes. Run a knife around the edges and carefully invert the loaf onto a cooling rack. Ensure that it is fully cooled before slicing.

Per Serving:
calories: 180 | fat: 3g | protein: 4g | carbs: 30g | fiber: 4g

Tea Scones

Prep time: 5 minutes | Cook time: 24 minutes | Makes 1 dozen scones

- ½ cup unsweetened plant-based milk
- 1 teaspoon apple cider vinegar
- 1 teaspoon pure vanilla extract
- 3 cups oat flour
- 2 tablespoons baking powder
- ½ cup date sugar (optional)
- ½ teaspoon salt (optional)
- ½ cup unsweetened applesauce
- ⅓ cup almond butter

1. Preheat the oven to 350°F (180°C) and line a baking sheet with parchment paper or a Silpat baking mat. 2. In a glass measuring cup, whisk together plant-based milk and apple cider vinegar. Let it sit for a few minutes to curdle, then add vanilla extract. 3. In a medium bowl, sift oat flour, baking powder, date sugar, and salt (if using). 4. In a small bowl, mix applesauce and almond butter using a fork. Use the fork to cut the applesauce mixture into the flour mixture until it becomes crumbly. Add the milk mixture and stir until just combined. Avoid overmixing. 5. Use a ¼-cup measuring cup or an ice-cream scoop to portion out the scone batter onto the prepared baking sheet. Lightly mist the measuring cup or scoop with water to help release the batter easily. Bake for 20 to 24 minutes, or until a knife inserted into the center comes out clean. 6. Allow the scones to cool on the baking sheet for a few minutes before transferring them to a cooling rack to cool completely.

Per Serving:
calories: 173 | fat: 5g | protein: 5g | carbs: 20g | fiber: 2g

Blueberry-Lime Sorbet

Prep time: 5 minutes | Cook time: 0 minutes | Serves 6

- 1 cup frozen blueberries
- 1 cup fresh blueberries
- 3 to 6 ice cubes
- ¼ cup unsweetened raisins
- 2 tablespoons lime juice

1. Using a high-efficiency blender, add the frozen blueberries, fresh blueberries, ice, raisins, and lime juice. Blend the ingredients for approximately 30 seconds, or until you achieve a smooth consistency. You may need to use the tamping tool to push the frozen ingredients towards the blades. 2. Once blended, serve the blueberry mixture immediately.

Per Serving:
calories: 116 | fat: 1g | protein: 2g | carbs: 30g | fiber: 4g

Nice Cream

Prep time: 10 minutes | Cook time: 0 minutes | Serves 2

2 cups frozen banana chunks
1 tablespoon soy milk
½ teaspoon vanilla extract

1. Place the bananas in a food processor and process them until they become crumbly. 2. Add the soy milk and vanilla to the food processor. Continue processing until the ingredients start to come together and resemble the texture of soft-serve ice cream. Serve immediately.

Per Serving:
calories: 112 | fat: 1g | protein: 2g | carbs: 28g | fiber: 3g

Blueberry Muffin Loaf

Prep time: 25 minutes | Cook time: 1 hour | Makes 1 loaf

Topping:
¼ cup maple sugar or coconut palm sugar (optional)
4 tablespoons whole spelt flour
Small pinch of fine sea salt (optional)
¼ teaspoon ground cinnamon
2 tablespoons coconut oil (optional)
Loaf:
⅓ cup unsweetened almond milk
1 tablespoon fresh orange juice
1½ cups whole spelt flour
½ cup almond flour
2 teaspoons aluminum-free baking powder
¼ teaspoon baking soda
½ teaspoon fine sea salt (optional)
1 teaspoon ground cinnamon
¼ cup unsweetened applesauce
⅓ cup coconut oil, plus extra for greasing the pan
⅓ cup plus 2 tablespoons maple sugar (optional)
1 teaspoon pure vanilla extract
1 cup fresh blueberries or frozen blueberries

1. Preheat the oven to 375°F (190°C). Lightly grease an 8- × 4-inch loaf pan with coconut oil. Line the pan with parchment paper, leaving an overhang on the two long sides, and set aside. 2. Make the Crumble Topping: In a small bowl, combine maple sugar, spelt flour, sea salt, cinnamon, and oil, if using. Lightly mix the topping with a fork until it starts clumping. Place the topping in the refrigerator while you make the loaf. 3. Make the Loaf: In a measuring cup, lightly whisk the almond milk with the orange juice, and set aside to curdle. 4. In a large bowl, whisk together the spelt flour, almond flour, baking powder, baking soda, sea salt, and cinnamon. Add the almond milk mixture to the flour mixture. Add the applesauce, oil, maple sugar, if using, and vanilla. Gently mix with a spatula until you have a unified batter, being careful not to overmix. 5. Gently fold the blueberries into the batter. Quickly scrape the batter into the prepared loaf pan, and top it with the crumble mixture. Gently press the crumble mixture into the surface of the loaf with your fingers. The crumble pieces should be surrounded by batter without being submerged. Slide the loaf pan into the oven, and bake for 55 to 60 minutes or until evenly browned on the top and a toothpick inserted into the center of the loaf comes out clean. 6. Cool the loaf completely in the pan before slicing and serving.

Per Serving: (⅛ loaf)
calories: 280 | fat: 11g | protein: 6g | carbs: 42g | fiber: 5g

Chocolate Pudding with Raspberries and Mint

Prep time: 20 minutes | Cook time: 20 minutes | Serves 4

1 (16-ounce / 454-g) package silken tofu
1 (15-ounce / 425-g) can full-fat coconut milk
5 tablespoons unsweetened cocoa powder
6 tablespoons maple syrup (optional)
1 tablespoon tapioca flour
1 tablespoon water
16 raspberries, for garnish
4 mint leaves, for garnish

1. In a blender, combine the tofu, coconut milk, cocoa powder, and maple syrup (if using) and purée until smooth. 2. Transfer the mixture to a medium saucepan set over medium heat and bring to a gentle boil. Lower the heat to medium. 3. In a small bowl, mix together the tapioca flour and water until smooth to make a slurry. Add the mixture to the saucepan and stir well until combined. Cook for an additional 2 to 3 minutes over medium heat, stirring constantly, to thicken the pudding. 4. Evenly divide the pudding among 4 cups or jars, cover, and refrigerate until chilled. The pudding will get firmer as it cools. 5. To serve, garnish each portion with 4 raspberries and 1 mint leaf. The pudding will last up to 4 days, covered, in the refrigerator.

Per Serving:
calories: 480 | fat: 29g | protein: 15g | carbs: 29g | fiber: 9g

Chocolate-Covered Strawberries

Prep time: 10 minutes | Cook time: 1 minute | Serves 20 strawberries

1 (12-ounce / 340-g) bag vegan semisweet chocolate chips
1 (1-pound / 454-g) carton strawberries, washed and dried

1. Prepare a baking sheet by lining it with parchment paper. 2. In a medium microwave-safe bowl, heat the chocolate chips in 30-second intervals, stirring between each time, until the chocolate is smooth and creamy. 3. Hold each strawberry by its stem and dip it into the melted chocolate, ensuring it is fully coated. Place the coated strawberry onto the prepared baking sheet. Repeat this process for all the strawberries. 4. Place the baking sheet in the refrigerator and let it chill for 20 to 25 minutes, or until the chocolate hardens. It is recommended to keep these strawberries refrigerated until you are ready to serve them.

Per Serving: (5 strawberries)
calories: 439 | fat: 25g | protein: 4g | carbs: 62g | fiber: 7g

Mango Sticky Rice

Prep time: 10 minutes | **Cook time:** 30 minutes | **Serves 6**

- 2½ cups water
- 1 cup short-grain brown rice
- ½ cup light or full-fat coconut milk
- 2 tablespoons coconut sugar (optional)
- 1 to 2 tablespoons fresh lime juice, to taste
- 2 mangos, peeled and diced
- Unsweetened shredded coconut (optional)

1. In a medium saucepan, bring water to a boil. Reduce the heat to medium-low and add the rice. Cook, stirring often, until the liquid is absorbed and the rice becomes tender, which usually takes about 30 minutes. 2. Remove the saucepan from the heat and stir in the coconut milk and sugar if desired. Add lime juice according to your taste preference. Transfer the cooked rice mixture into a shallow glass dish. Top it with mango slices and garnish with coconut if desired. Serve immediately. (Alternatively, you can refrigerate the dish and serve it cold, but remember to garnish with coconut just before serving.)

Per Serving:
calories: 244 | fat: 5g | protein: 4g | carbs: 47g | fiber: 3g

No-Bake Mocha Cheesecake

Prep time: 15 minutes | **Cook time:** 10 minutes | **Makes 1 cake**

Crust:
- 12 chocolate sandwich cookies

Filling:
- 1 (13½-ounce / 383-g) can full-fat coconut milk
- 1 tablespoon agar flakes
- 1 tablespoon plus 1 teaspoon instant coffee
- ¼ cup maple syrup (optional)
- ¼ cup water
- ½ teaspoon vanilla extract
- 1 cup raw cashews, soaked in hot water for at least 10 minutes, and drained
- 2 tablespoons unsweetened cocoa powder

1. To make the crust, place the cookies in a food processor and pulse until they are roughly chopped. Continue processing until they resemble crumbs. Transfer the crumbs to a 9-inch pie plate and press them down to form a crust. Put it in the freezer while you prepare the filling. 2. For the filling, separate the solids from the coconut milk and transfer them to a high-speed blender. Pour the liquid into a small saucepan. Don't worry if some of the solids end up in the saucepan; they will melt.
3. In the saucepan with the liquids, add agar, coffee, maple syrup (if desired), water, and vanilla. Whisk everything together to combine. Place the saucepan over medium heat and let the mixture come to a simmer, with small bubbles breaking the surface. Cook for 3 minutes, whisking frequently, until the agar is completely dissolved.
4. Add cashews and cocoa to the blender with the coconut milk solids. Process everything until smooth, pausing as needed to scrape down the sides of the blender.
5. With the blender running on low speed, slowly pour in the contents of the saucepan. Continue processing until the filling is smooth and well combined. Pour the filling into the prepared crust and refrigerate until set, at least 30 minutes. Serve chilled.

Per Serving: (⅛ cake)
calories: 325 | fat: 23g | protein: 5g | carbs: 29g | fiber: 3g

Two-Minute Turtles

Prep time: 5 minutes | **Cook time:** 0 minutes | **Makes 12 turtles**

- 12 pitted dates
- 12 toasted pecans
- ¼ cup chocolate chips

1. Make a lengthwise slit in each date, being careful not to cut all the way through. Gently widen the opening and insert 1 pecan and a few chocolate chips into each date. 2. Repeat the process with the remaining dates, pecans, and chocolate chips. Serve immediately. The stuffed dates can be stored in an airtight container for up to 2 days.

Per Serving: (2 turtles)
calories: 95 | fat: 41g | protein: 16g | carbs: 2g | fiber: 2g

Gooey Bittersweet Chocolate Pudding Cake

Prep time: 15 minutes | **Cook time:** 3 to 4 hours | **Serves 6 to 8**

Cake:
- 1 cup whole-wheat flour
- ¼ cup cocoa powder
- 2 teaspoons baking powder
- ½ teaspoon ground cinnamon
- ¼ teaspoon salt (optional)
- ⅓ cup unsweetened applesauce
- 2 teaspoons vanilla extract
- ⅔ cup unsweetened vanilla or plain plant-based milk
- 2 tablespoons date syrup or maple syrup (optional)
- Nonstick cooking spray (optional)

Pudding:
- ¼ cup cocoa powder
- 1 teaspoon instant coffee
- ½ cup date syrup or maple syrup (optional)
- 1 teaspoon vanilla extract
- 1 cup hot water

1. Prepare the cake: In a medium bowl, whisk together flour, cocoa powder, baking powder, cinnamon, and salt (if using). 2. In another medium bowl, whisk together applesauce, vanilla, milk, and date syrup (if using). Pour the applesauce mixture into the flour mixture and stir until just combined. Be careful not to overmix. 3. Grease the inside of the slow cooker with cooking spray (if using) or line it with a slow cooker liner. Pour the cake batter into the slow cooker and spread it evenly on the bottom.
4. Prepare the pudding: In a medium bowl, whisk together cocoa powder, coffee, date syrup (if using), vanilla, and hot water. Pour the mixture over the cake batter in the slow cooker. It will appear watery. 5. Cover the slow cooker and cook on Low for 3 to 4 hours. The cake will be ready when the top looks dry and it has achieved a pudding-like texture underneath. Serve immediately for the best results.

Per Serving:
calories: 195 | fat: 2g | protein: 4g | carbs: 44g | fiber: 4g

Coconut Chia Pudding

Prep time: 5 minutes | Cook time: 0 minutes | Makes 3 cups

1 pound (454 g) raw young coconut meat, defrosted if frozen, any liquid reserved
1¼ cups unpasteurized coconut water
1 tablespoon vanilla extract
6 tablespoons chia seeds

1. Put the coconut meat (and any liquid that accumulated as it defrosted, if frozen) in an upright blender. Add the coconut water and vanilla and blend on high speed until completely smooth. Pour into a widemouthed quart jar or a medium bowl, add the chia seeds, and whisk thoroughly, making sure there are no clumps of seeds hiding anywhere. Allow to sit for a few minutes and then whisk again. Leave the whisk in place and refrigerate for at least 1 hour, or until completely chilled, whisking every now and then to distribute the chia seeds evenly. The pudding will thicken further overnight; if it gets too thick, stir in a splash of water, coconut water, or nut milk. Store the pudding in an airtight glass jar or other container in the fridge for up to 3 days.

Per Serving: (½ cup)

calories: 296 | fat: 26g | protein: 3g | carbs: 15g | fiber: 8g

Apple Crisp

Prep time: 10 minutes | Cook time: 50 minutes | Serves 6 to 8

Filling:
3 pounds (1.4 kg) Granny Smith apples (about 8 apples), peeled, cored, and cut into ¼-inch slices
2 tablespoons cornstarch
1 teaspoon ground cinnamon
½ teaspoon ground ginger
⅛ teaspoon ground cloves
½ cup 100% pure maple syrup (optional)

Topping:
¼ cup 100% pure maple syrup (optional)
3 tablespoons cashew butter
2 tablespoons unsweetened applesauce
1 teaspoon pure vanilla extract
1½ cup rolled oats
½ teaspoon ground cinnamon
¼ teaspoon salt (optional)

1. Preheat the oven to 400°F (205°C). Line an 8 × 8-inch pan with parchment paper, ensuring that it covers the sides of the pan, or have an 8 × 8-inch nonstick or silicone baking pan ready. Prepare the Filling: 2. In a large mixing bowl, place the apples. 3. Sprinkle cornstarch, cinnamon, ginger, and cloves over the apple slices. Toss well to coat them evenly. Pour maple syrup (if using) over the mixture and stir to combine. Transfer the apple mixture into the prepared baking pan. Prepare the Topping:
4. In a small bowl, use a fork to mix together maple syrup (if using), cashew butter, applesauce, and vanilla until relatively smooth. Add oats, cinnamon, and salt (if using), and toss to coat. Assemble the Crisp:
5. Spread the topping over the apple mixture. Place the pan in the preheated oven and bake for 20 minutes. Then, reduce the oven temperature to 350°F (180°C) and continue baking for an additional 30 minutes, or until the topping turns golden and the filling is bubbling. 6. Remove the pan from the oven and place it on a cooling rack. Serve the crisp while warm.

Per Serving:

calories: 232 | fat: 4g | protein: 4g | carbs: 45g | fiber: 8g

Peanut Butter Nice Cream

Prep time: 5 minutes | Cook time: 0 minutes | Serves 2

3 frozen ripe bananas, broken into thirds
3 tablespoons plant-based milk
2 tablespoons defatted peanut powder
1 teaspoon vanilla extract

1. In a food processor, combine the bananas, milk, peanut powder, and vanilla. 2. Process on medium speed for 30 to 60 seconds, or until the bananas have been blended into a smooth soft-serve consistency, and serve.

Per Serving:

calories: 237 | fat: 3g | protein: 10g | carbs: 45g | fiber: 7g

Superfood Caramels

Prep time: 10 minutes | Cook time: 10 minutes | Makes 12 pieces

12 to 14 Medjool dates, pitted
½ cup raw tahini
1 tablespoon lucuma powder
1 teaspoon Himalayan pink salt, plus more for sprinkling (optional)
1 (80-g) bar dark organic chocolate

1. In a food processor, combine dates, tahini, lucuma, and salt (if using). Blend until well mixed, and the mixture starts to form a ball in the food processor. 2. Transfer the "caramel" mixture onto a piece of parchment paper and cover it with another piece. Use a rolling pin to flatten it into a square or rectangular shape, about ½ inch thick. Place it in the freezer for at least 20 minutes, or until firm enough to cut. 3. Leave the caramel in the freezer and line a large plate with parchment paper near your stovetop. 4. In a double boiler or a heat-safe medium bowl set over a saucepan with boiling water, gently melt the chocolate over low heat. Stir occasionally to prevent overheating. Once fully melted, reduce the heat or turn it off. Take the caramels out of the freezer and place them on a cutting board. Cut them into square or rectangular pieces, similar in size to regular caramels. 5. Using a spoon, carefully dip each caramel into the melted chocolate, ensuring it is fully coated. Place the coated caramel on the parchment-lined plate. 6. Sprinkle Himalayan pink salt (if using) over the coated caramel before the chocolate hardens. Repeat this process with the remaining pieces. Then, place the entire plate in the freezer. 7. After the chocolate has hardened for at least 30 minutes, enjoy some pieces immediately. Store the rest in an airtight container in the freezer.

Per Serving:

calories: 163 | fat: 7g | protein: 3g | carbs: 23g | fiber: 3g

Nilla Cookies

Prep time: 5 minutes | Cook time: 10 minutes | Makes 36 cookies

⅔ cup unsweetened plant-based milk
¼ cup almond butter
¼ cup unsweetened applesauce
⅔ cup date sugar (optional)
1 teaspoon pure vanilla extract
1 vanilla bean, halved
1 cup oat flour
⅔ cup coconut flour
1 tablespoon cornstarch
2 teaspoons baking powder
½ teaspoon salt (optional)

1. Preheat the oven to 350ºF (180ºC). Line 2 large baking sheets with parchment paper or Silpat baking mats. 2. In a large mixing bowl, use a strong fork to beat together the plant-based milk, almond butter, applesauce, and date sugar (if using). Once relatively smooth, mix in the vanilla. Scrape the seeds from the vanilla bean and add to the batter. Mix well. 3. Add in the oat flour, coconut flour, cornstarch, baking powder, and salt (if using). Mix well. The dough will be stiff. 4. Roll the dough into walnut-size balls and place them on the prepared baking sheets, a little over an inch apart. Flatten the cookies a bit, so that they resemble thick discs (they don't spread much at all during baking). Bake for 8 to 10 minutes. The longer you bake them, the crispier they will be. 5. Remove the cookies from the oven and let them cool on the baking sheets for 5 minutes, and then transfer to a cooling rack to cool completely.

Per Serving:
calories: 80 | fat: 2g | protein: 2g | carbs: 12g | fiber: 1g

Gluten-Free Vegan Waffles

Prep time: 15 minutes | Cook time: 15 minutes | Makes 8 waffles

1¼ cups unsweetened almond milk
2 tablespoons plus 2 teaspoons ground flaxseeds
½ cup almond flour
1 cup gluten-free oat flour
½ cup millet flour
¼ cup brown rice flour
1 tablespoon aluminum-free baking powder
½ cup mashed bananas or ½ cup mashed squash
¼ cup melted extra-virgin coconut oil, plus more for the waffle iron (optional)
1 tablespoon vanilla extract
1 teaspoon raw apple cider vinegar

1. Whisk the almond milk and ground flaxseeds together in a medium bowl. Set aside for at least 10 minutes to thicken. 2. Preheat the waffle iron. Meanwhile, put the almond flour in a medium bowl and break up any lumps with your fingertips. Sift in the oat flour, millet flour, brown rice flour, and baking powder and whisk to combine; set aside. Whisk the flax mixture again, add the bananas or squash, oil, vanilla, and vinegar, and stir well. Add the flour mixture and stir with a rubber spatula until just combined. Lightly brush the waffle iron with oil and scoop about a scant ½ cup batter (the exact amount will depend on your iron) onto the iron. Cook until golden; vegan waffles usually need to cook for a few minutes longer than suggested for regular waffles. Remove the waffles and serve immediately with any of the toppings suggested, or place on a rack to cool if you are making them ahead. Repeat with the remaining batter. To store, once the waffles are cool, transfer to airtight containers and refrigerate for up to 3 days or freeze for up to 3 months.

Per Serving: (1 waffle)
calories: 193 | fat: 10g | protein: 4g | carbs: 23g | fiber: 2g

Stone Fruit Chia Pudding

Prep time: 10 minutes | Cook time: 10 minutes | Makes 3 cups

1¼ pounds (567 g) stone fruit, halved, pitted, and cut into 1-inch dice
¾ cup freshly squeezed orange juice or ½ cup filtered water
Pinch of fine sea salt (optional)
½ cup raw cashews or macadamia nuts
2 tablespoons coconut butter
1 teaspoon vanilla extract
¼ cup chia seeds

1. Combine the fruit, orange juice, and salt, if using, in a medium pot and bring to a boil over high heat. Cover, reduce the heat to low, and simmer for 8 to 10 minutes, until the fruit has cooked through. Remove from the heat and allow to cool slightly. 2. Transfer the mixture to an upright blender, add the cashews, coconut butter, and vanilla, and blend until completely smooth. Pour into a widemouthed quart jar or a medium bowl, add the chia seeds, and whisk thoroughly, making sure there are no clumps of seeds hiding anywhere. Allow to sit for a few minutes and then whisk again. Leave the whisk in place and refrigerate for at least 1 hour, or until completely chilled, whisking every now and then to distribute the chia seeds evenly and to help cool the pudding quickly. The pudding will thicken further overnight; if it gets too thick, stir in a splash of water or nut milk. Store the pudding in an airtight glass jar or other container in the fridge for up to 5 days.

Per Serving: (½ cup)
calories: 199 | fat: 15g | protein: 3g | carbs: 17g | fiber: 5g

Sweet Potato and Chocolate Pudding

Prep time: 10 minutes | Cook time: 0 minutes | Serves 4

2 cups cooked sweet potato, cooled
1 cup pitted dates
¾ cup unsweetened soy milk
6 tablespoons cocoa powder
1½ teaspoons vanilla extract

1. In a high-efficiency blender, combine the sweet potato, dates, soy milk, cocoa powder, and vanilla. Blend until smooth, using a tamper accessory if necessary. Refrigerate in an airtight container until ready to serve.

Per Serving:
calories: 263 | fat: 2g | protein: 6g | carbs: 62g | fiber: 10g

Black Sesame-Ginger Quick Bread

Prep time: 20 minutes | Cook time: 50 minutes | Make 12 muffins

⅔ cup black sesame seeds
1 cup candied ginger
1½ cups plus 2 tablespoons whole wheat pastry flour
1 cup almond meal
2½ teaspoons baking powder
½ teaspoon salt (optional)
¾ cup almond milk, room temperature
¾ cup coconut sugar (optional)
½ cup melted coconut oil (optional)
2 tablespoons chia seeds
1 tablespoon fresh lemon juice
1 tablespoon ginger juice

1. Adjust an oven rack to the middle position, and preheat the oven to 350°F (180°C). Line two muffin pans with liners. 2. Pulse the sesame seeds in a food processor until ground. Transfer to a large bowl and set aside. 3. Add the ginger and 2 tablespoons of the flour to the food processor; pulse until the ginger is roughly chopped. (The flour will help keep it suspended in the batter as it bakes.) 4. Add the remaining flour, almond meal, baking powder, and salt (if desired) to the bowl with the ground sesame seeds. Stir to combine, then stir in the ginger. Make a well in the center. 5. Process the almond milk, sugar, coconut oil (if desired), chia seeds, lemon juice, and ginger juice in the now-empty food processor until completely combined. Transfer to the bowl with the dry ingredients and gently fold in the wet ingredients until just combined. (The batter will be quite thick.) 6. Scoop the batter into the muffin pans. Smooth the tops with a wet spatula. Bake for 30 minutes, until a toothpick inserted in the center comes out clean. 7. Allow to cool for 10 minutes in the pans, then allow to cool completely on a rack before slicing or peeling off the liners.

Per Serving: (2 muffins)
calories: 449 | fat: 30g | protein: 9g | carbs: 42g | fiber: 6g

Coconut Crumble Bars

Prep time: 10 minutes | Cook time: 15 minutes | Makes 8 bars

2 cups raw and unsalted almonds
10 pitted dates
2 scoops soy protein isolate, chocolate flavor
½ cup cocoa powder
½ cup shredded coconut

1. Preheat the oven to 257°F (125°C) and line a baking sheet with parchment paper. 2. Put the almonds on the baking sheet and roast them for about 10 to 15 minutes or until they're fragrant. 3. Meanwhile, cover the dates with water in a small bowl and let them sit for about 10 minutes. Drain the dates after soaking and make sure no water is left. 4. Add the almonds, dates, chocolate protein and cocoa powder to a food processor and blend into a chunky mixture. 5. Alternatively, add all ingredients to a medium bowl, cover it, and process using a handheld blender. 6. Line a loaf pan with parchment paper. Add the almond mixture to the loaf pan, spread it out and press it down firmly until it's 1-inch-thick (2.5 cm) all over. 7. Add the shredded coconut in an even layer on top and press it down firmly to make it stick. 8. Divide into 8 bars, serve cold and enjoy! 9. Store the bars in an airtight container in the fridge, and consume within 6 days. Alternatively, store in the freezer for a maximum of 90 days.

Per Serving:
calories: 301 | fat: 21g | protein: 17g | carbs: 9g | fiber: 5g

Chapter 6: Vegetables and Sides

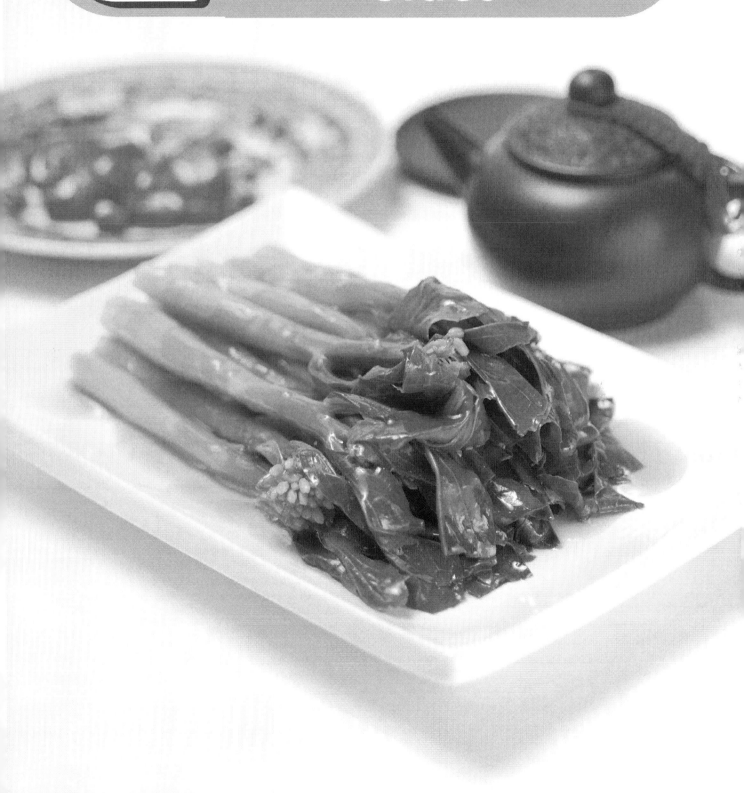

Garlic Mashed Potatoes

Prep time: 15 minutes | Cook time: 3 to 4 hours | Serves 4 to 6

6 russet potatoes (about 3 pounds / 1.4 kg), peeled
1 cup store-bought low-sodium vegetable broth
1 cup unsweetened plant-based milk, plus more for mashing
5 to 6 garlic cloves, minced
Ground black pepper
Salt (optional)

1. Cut the potatoes into 1- to 2-inch cubes and place them in the slow cooker. Pour in the broth. 2. Cover the slow cooker and cook on High for 3 to 4 hours or on Low for 8 hours, until the potatoes are tender and can be easily mashed. 3. Add the milk and garlic to the cooked potatoes and mash them to your desired consistency. You may need to add up to ½ cup more milk, depending on how creamy you prefer your mashed potatoes. Season with generous amounts of pepper and salt (if using). Serve and enjoy.

Per Serving:
calories: 286 | fat: 1g | protein: 8g | carbs: 64g | fiber: 5g

Yellow Bell Pepper Boats

Prep time: 30 minutes | Cook time: 50 minutes | Serves 6

Bell Pepper Boats:
2 medium potatoes, halved
1 ear corn, kernels removed (about ½ cup)
½ small onion, peeled and finely chopped
1 small green bell pepper, seeded and finely chopped (about ¼ cup)
¼ teaspoon grated ginger
½ clove garlic, peeled and minced
½ teaspoon minced serrano chile, or to taste (for less heat, remove the seeds)
½ teaspoon salt, or to taste
(optional)
1 teaspoon fresh lime juice
2 yellow bell peppers
¼ cup sunflower seeds, toasted
Hot Sauce:
1 large tomato, chopped (about 2 cups)
½ teaspoon cayenne pepper
½ teaspoon salt, or to taste (optional)
½ clove garlic, peeled and mashed to a paste
½ tablespoon finely chopped cilantro

Make the Bell Pepper Boats:
1. Preheat the oven to 350°F (180°C). 2. In a saucepan, boil the potatoes in water over medium heat for about 15 minutes until they are tender. Remove from heat, drain, and let them cool. Mash the potatoes in a mixing bowl. 3. In a small pan, combine corn and 1 cup of water. Cook on medium heat until the corn is tender, approximately 5 to 7 minutes. Drain the corn and add it to the mashed potatoes along with the onion, green pepper, ginger, garlic, serrano chile, salt (if using), and lime juice. Mix everything well. 4. Cut the yellow peppers into boat shapes by slicing them into three long pieces each. Remove the seeds. Fill each pepper slice with the potato mixture and sprinkle with sunflower seeds. Cover and bake for 30 to 35 minutes until the yellow peppers become soft when pierced with a fork.
Make the Hot Sauce:
5. Blend the tomato in a blender until smooth. Transfer the puree to a saucepan and add cayenne pepper, salt (if using), and garlic. Bring the mixture to a boil and cook for 5 minutes. Reduce the heat to low and simmer for an additional 5 minutes. 6. To serve, spread the hot sauce on top of the baked bell peppers. Garnish with cilantro.

Per Serving:
calories: 138 | fat: 3g | protein: 4g | carbs: 25g | fiber: 4g

Savory Sweet Potato Casserole

Prep time: 15 minutes | Cook time: 30 minutes | Serves 6

8 cooked sweet potatoes
½ cup vegetable broth
1 tablespoon dried sage
1 teaspoon dried thyme
1 teaspoon dried rosemary

1. Preheat your oven to 375°F (190°C). 2. After cooking the sweet potatoes, peel and discard the skin. Place the cooked sweet potatoes in a baking dish and mash them using a fork or potato masher. Add the broth, sage, thyme, and rosemary, and mix everything together. 3. Bake the mixture in the oven for 30 minutes, then it's ready to be served.

Per Serving:
calories: 154 | fat: 0g | protein: 3g | carbs: 35g | fiber: 6g

Zucchini "Parmesan"

Prep time: 10 minutes | Cook time: 20 minutes | Serves 4

4 zucchini, sliced into ½-inch rounds
½ cup almond milk
1 teaspoon arrowroot powder
1 teaspoon fresh lemon juice
½ teaspoon salt (optional)
½ cup whole wheat bread crumbs
¼ cup hemp seeds
¼ cup nutritional yeast
½ teaspoon garlic powder
¼ teaspoon black pepper
¼ teaspoon crushed red pepper

1. Preheat your oven to 375°F (190°C) and line two baking sheets with parchment paper. 2. In a medium bowl, combine the zucchini, almond milk, arrowroot powder, lemon juice, and ¼ teaspoon of salt (if desired). Stir well to combine. 3. In a large bowl with a lid, mix together the bread crumbs, hemp seeds, nutritional yeast, garlic powder, black pepper, and crushed red pepper. Add the zucchini slices in batches and shake until they are evenly coated with the mixture. 4. Arrange the coated zucchini slices in a single layer on the prepared baking sheets. Bake for approximately 20 minutes, or until the zucchini slices turn golden brown. Serve and enjoy.

Per Serving:
calories: 191 | fat: 6g | protein: 11g | carbs: 25g | fiber: 5g

Stir-Fried Vegetables with Miso and Sake

Prep time: 25 minutes | **Cook time:** 10 minutes | **Serves 4**

¼ cup mellow white miso
½ cup vegetable stock, or low-sodium vegetable broth
¼ cup sake
1 medium yellow onion, peeled and thinly sliced
1 large carrot, peeled, cut in half lengthwise, and then cut into half-moons on the diagonal
1 medium red bell pepper, seeded and cut into ½-inch strips
1 large head broccoli, cut into florets
½ pound (227 g) snow peas, trimmed
2 cloves garlic, peeled and minced
½ cup chopped cilantro (optional)
Salt and freshly ground black pepper, to taste

1. In a small bowl, whisk together the miso, vegetable stock, and sake, then set the mixture aside. 2. Heat a large skillet over high heat. Add the onion, carrot, red pepper, and broccoli, and stir-fry for 4 to 5 minutes. To prevent sticking, add water 1 to 2 tablespoons at a time. Next, add the snow peas and continue stir-frying for an additional 4 minutes. Stir in the garlic and cook for 30 seconds. 3. Pour the miso mixture into the skillet and cook until everything is heated through. Remove the pan from the heat, and if desired, add the cilantro for added flavor. Finally, season the stir-fried vegetables with salt and pepper to taste.

Per Serving:
calories: 135 | fat: 1g | protein: 7g | carbs: 24g | fiber: 7g

Sautéed Root Vegetables with Parsley, Poppy Seeds, and Lemon

Prep time: 10 minutes | **Cook time:** 10 minutes | **Serves 4**

2 tablespoons extra-virgin coconut oil (optional)
2 large garlic cloves, finely chopped
1 pound (454 g) root vegetables, grated
1 teaspoon fine sea salt, plus more to taste (optional)
1 tablespoon poppy seeds
Grated zest of 1 small lemon
1 tablespoon freshly squeezed lemon juice
1½ cups fresh flat-leaf parsley leaves, coarsely chopped

1. In a large skillet, heat the oil over medium heat. Add the garlic and sauté until it turns golden, about 1 minute. Stir in the grated vegetables and add salt if desired. Cook for 8 minutes or until the vegetables become soft. 2. Remove the skillet from the heat and mix in the poppy seeds, lemon zest, lemon juice, and parsley. Taste and season with more salt if needed. Serve the dish warm or at room temperature. Leftovers can be stored in an airtight container in the refrigerator for up to 3 days.

Per Serving:
calories: 130 | fat: 8g | protein: 2g | carbs: 14g | fiber: 4g

Teriyaki Mushrooms

Prep time: 15 minutes | **Cook time:** 2 hours | **Serves 4 to 6**

2 (8-ounce / 227-g) packages whole cremini mushrooms
½ cup low-sodium soy sauce, tamari, or coconut aminos
¼ cup maple syrup (optional)
2 tablespoons rice vinegar
2 garlic cloves, minced
1 piece (1-inch) fresh ginger, peeled and minced, or 1 teaspoon ground ginger
2 tablespoons sesame seeds, divided
2 scallions, green and white parts, chopped, for serving

1. Place the mushrooms in the slow cooker. 2. In a measuring cup or medium bowl, mix together soy sauce, maple syrup (if using), rice vinegar, garlic, and ginger. Pour the sauce over the mushrooms and sprinkle with 1 tablespoon of sesame seeds. Cover the slow cooker and cook on High for 2 hours or on Low for 4 hours.
3. Serve the cooked mushrooms garnished with scallions and the remaining 1 tablespoon of sesame seeds.

Per Serving:
calories: 129 | fat: 3g | protein: 7g | carbs: 21g | fiber: 2g

Spicy Butternut Squash Bisque

Prep time: 10 minutes | **Cook time:** 30 minutes | **Serves 4**

Olive oil cooking spray
1 large butternut squash, peeled, seeded and cut into 1-inch cubes (about 3 cups)
2 garlic cloves, peeled
1 teaspoon smoked paprika
½ teaspoon salt (optional)
4 cups unsweetened plant-based milk
2 tablespoons nutritional yeast
2 tablespoons tomato paste
1 teaspoon sriracha
4 tablespoons chopped cilantro leaves, for garnish
4 tablespoons plain plant-based yogurt, for garnish
4 tablespoons pepitas, for garnish (optional)

1. Preheat your oven to 400ºF (205ºC) and lightly grease a sheet pan with olive oil cooking spray. 2. Place the squash, garlic, smoked paprika, and salt (if preferred) on the prepared sheet pan. Toss everything together until the squash is evenly coated. Roast in the oven for 10 minutes. Then, using a spatula, flip the squash pieces and continue baking for another 10 minutes or until they are cooked through. 3. Once the squash and garlic are roasted, transfer them to a blender. Add the plant-based milk, nutritional yeast, tomato paste, and sriracha. Blend the mixture until it turns smooth and creamy. Pour the blended soup into a large saucepan and heat over medium heat until warmed through. Taste the soup and adjust the seasonings to your liking.
4. Divide the soup into four bowls and garnish each serving with 1 tablespoon of cilantro, yogurt, and pepitas. Serve and enjoy your flavorful roasted squash soup!

Per Serving:
calories: 141 | fat: 3g | protein: 8g | carbs: 24g | fiber: 3g

Vegan Goulash

Prep time: 20 minutes | **Cook time:** 50 minutes | **Serves 5**

5 tablespoons olive oil (optional)	½ cup dry red wine
12 medium onions, finely chopped	3 to 6 cups vegetable broth
1 head garlic, minced	10 medium potatoes, skinned, cubed
4 red bell peppers, cored and chopped	1 (7-ounce / 198-g) pack tempeh
10 small tomatoes, cubed	Salt and pepper to taste (optional)
4 tablespoons paprika powder	¼ cup fresh parsley, chopped

1. In a large pot over medium heat, heat the olive oil. Sauté the onions until they turn brown. Add the minced garlic and stir for 1 minute. Then, add the chopped bell peppers and continue to cook, stirring, for another 3 minutes. Next, blend in the tomatoes, paprika powder, salt (if desired), pepper, and dry red wine. Stir well and let the mixture cook for an additional 2 minutes. Add the vegetable broth and potato cubes to the pot, stirring to combine all the ingredients. Cover the pot with a lid and let the goulash cook for another 5 minutes. 2. Reduce the heat to low and gently cook the goulash for 15 minutes. The goulash will thicken, and the potatoes will cook properly. Add the tempeh and taste to see if the goulash needs more salt and pepper. Allow the goulash to cook for another 15 minutes. Test the potatoes with a fork to check if they have softened. If the potatoes are still hard, cook the mixture for a few more minutes until they become tender. Once the potatoes are soft, stir in the parsley and take the goulash off the heat. 3. Let the goulash cool down for about 10 minutes and serve, or refrigerate it for a longer period if desired.

Per Serving:
calories: 591 | fat: 18g | protein: 16g | carbs: 74g | fiber: 14g

Fennel and Cherry Tomato Gratin

Prep time: 15 minutes | **Cook time:** 55 minutes | **Serves 6**

2 fennel bulbs, long fronds and top stalks trimmed off	(optional)
1 cup whole cherry tomatoes	Topping:
⅓ cup vegetable stock	½ cup raw pine nuts
2 tablespoons dry white wine	½ cup raw walnut halves
1 tablespoon virgin olive oil (optional)	1 tablespoon virgin olive oil
2 teaspoons minced fresh thyme leaves	1 tablespoon nutritional yeast
Salt and pepper, to taste	½ teaspoon garlic powder
	2 teaspoons minced fresh thyme leaves

1. Preheat your oven to 375°F (190°C). 2. Cut the fennel bulbs into 2-inch wedges, ensuring to remove any tough pieces of the core. Arrange the fennel wedges facing up in a 13- × 9-inch glass or metal baking dish. 3. Place the tomatoes in the spaces between the fennel wedges in the dish. Carefully pour the vegetable stock and white wine into the pan, ensuring even distribution. Drizzle the olive oil over the fennel wedges. Season the fennel with minced thyme, and add salt and pepper if desired. Cover the dish tightly with foil and bake in the oven for 35 minutes. 4. While the gratin bakes, prepare the topping. In a food processor, combine the pine nuts, walnut halves, olive oil, nutritional yeast, garlic powder, and minced thyme. Pulse the mixture until it forms a crumbly topping that holds together in small chunks.
5. After 35 minutes of baking, remove the fennel from the oven and take off the foil. Sprinkle the prepared topping all over the surface. Place the gratin back into the oven, uncovered, and bake for another 20 minutes or until the topping turns golden brown, and the fennel becomes fork-tender. Serve the gratin hot.

Per Serving:
calories: 196 | fat: 16g | protein: 5g | carbs: 10g | fiber: 4g

Ratatouille

Prep time: 30 minutes | **Cook time:** 25 minutes | **Serves 4**

1 medium red onion, peeled and diced	1 small zucchini, diced
1 medium red bell pepper, seeded and diced	4 cloves garlic, peeled and minced
1 medium eggplant, about 1 pound / 454 g, stemmed and diced	½ cup chopped basil
	1 large tomato, diced
	Salt and freshly ground black pepper, to taste

1. Place the onion in a medium saucepan and sauté over medium heat for 10 minutes. Add water 1 to 2 tablespoons at a time to keep the onions from sticking to the pan. Add the red pepper, eggplant, zucchini, and garlic. Cook, covered, for 15 minutes, stirring occasionally. 2. Stir in the basil and tomatoes, and season with salt and pepper.

Per Serving:
calories: 34 | fat: 0g | protein: 1g | carbs: 7g | fiber: 2g

Sheet-Pan Garlicky Kale

Prep time: 5 minutes | **Cook time:** 15 minutes | **Serves 2**

2 garlic cloves, minced	¼ teaspoon salt (optional)
2 teaspoons extra-virgin olive oil (optional)	¼ teaspoon black pepper
1 bunch kale, roughly chopped	¼ teaspoon garlic powder

1. Preheat the oven to 400°F (205°C). 2. In a large bowl, combine the garlic, olive oil, kale, salt (if using), black pepper, and garlic powder and toss until well combined. Spread out the kale on a sheet pan and bake for 10 minutes. Using a spatula, turn the kale and continue to cook for another 5 minutes, until the kale is wilted and bright green.

Per Serving:
calories: 144 | fat: 6g | protein: 9g | carbs: 19g | fiber: 7g

Ultimate Veggie Wrap with Kale Pesto

Prep time: 20 minutes | Cook time: 10 minutes | Serves 2

Kale Pesto:
¼ cup raw cashews, soaked at least 2 hours
1 cup kale, de-stemmed and coarsely chopped
1 clove garlic
½ teaspoon salt (optional)
2 tablespoons nutritional yeast
3 tablespoons extra virgin olive oil (optional)
Wrap:
½ cup broccoli florets
2 spinach tortillas
¼ cup grated carrots
¼ cup diced red onion
½ yellow bell pepper, diced
6 ounces (170 g) spinach
2 tablespoons raw shelled hempseed
2 tablespoons sunflower seed kernels

Make Kale Pesto:
1. In a small food processor, combine cashews, kale, garlic, and salt (if desired). Process for about 30 seconds until well blended. Add nutritional yeast and oil, then process for a few more seconds until the mixture is smooth. Set aside.
Assemble:
2. Fill a medium saucepan with water and place a steamer insert inside. Bring the water to a boil. Add broccoli to the steamer insert and steam over boiling water for 10 minutes. Remove the broccoli from the steamer and set it aside. 3. Lay out the spinach tortillas. Divide the kale pesto between the two tortillas and spread it evenly, leaving about 1 inch of space around all edges. Divide the remaining ingredients in half and place each half next to each other down the length of each tortilla. 4. Roll up each tortilla snugly, being careful not to tear them. Cut each tortilla in half and serve.

Per Serving:
calories: 554 | fat: 36g | protein: 24g | carbs: 34g | fiber: 8g

Vegetable Spring Rolls with Spicy Peanut Dipping Sauce

Prep time: 15 minutes | Cook time: 10 minutes | Serves 2

Spicy Peanut Dipping Sauce:
2 tablespoons defatted peanut powder
1 tablespoon maple syrup (optional)
1 tablespoon rice vinegar
½ teaspoon onion powder
½ teaspoon garlic powder
½ teaspoon red pepper flakes
Spring Rolls:
6 rice paper wraps
6 large lettuce leaves
1½ cups cooked brown rice
1 cup shredded carrots
1 bunch fresh cilantro
1 bunch fresh mint
1 bunch fresh basil

Make Spicy Peanut Dipping Sauce:
1. In a small saucepan over medium heat, combine the peanut powder, maple syrup (if desired), rice vinegar, onion powder, garlic powder, and red pepper flakes. Cook for 10 minutes, stirring occasionally. Remove the sauce from the heat, and set aside to cool. Make Spring Rolls: 1. Fill a shallow bowl or pan with warm water, and dip a rice paper wrap in the water for 10 to 15 seconds. Remove and place on a cutting board or other clean, smooth surface. 2. Lay a lettuce leaf down flat on a rice paper wrap, then add ¼ cup of brown rice, 2 to 3 tablespoons of shredded carrots, and a few leaves each of cilantro, mint, and basil. 3. Wrap the sides of the rice paper halfway into the center, then roll the wrap from the bottom to the top to form a tight roll. 4. Repeat for the remaining spring rolls. Serve with the sauce in a dipping bowl on the side.

Per Serving:
calories: 263 | fat: 3g | protein: 11g | carbs: 46g | fiber: 5g

Spring Steamed Vegetables with Savory Goji Berry Cream

Prep time: 15 minutes | Cook time: 10 minutes | Serves 6

Savory Goji Berry Cream:
¼ cup dried goji berries
1 tablespoon apple cider vinegar
1 tablespoon mellow or light miso
1 tablespoon fresh lemon juice
1 (1-inch) piece of fresh ginger, peeled and chopped
1 teaspoon pure maple syrup (optional)
3 tablespoons virgin olive oil
(optional)
Salt and pepper, to taste (optional)
Vegetables:
1½ pounds (680 g) trimmed spring vegetables
Salt and pepper, to taste (optional)
Garnishes:
Scant ¼ cup walnut halves, toasted and chopped
1 green onion, thinly sliced

1. Prepare the Savory Goji Berry Cream: Place the goji berries in a small bowl and pour boiling water over them. Allow the berries to sit for 5 minutes until they plump up and become soft. Transfer the goji berries to a blender, but remember to keep the soaking water. 2. To the blender, add apple cider vinegar, miso, lemon juice, ginger, maple syrup, olive oil, salt, and pepper if desired. Pour in 3 tablespoons of the goji soaking water. Blend the mixture on high speed until it becomes creamy and smooth. Set the savory goji berry cream aside. 3. Prepare the Vegetables: Trim the vegetables as needed and place a large pot with about 1 inch of water on the stove. Bring the water to a simmer. Arrange the vegetables in a steamer basket and place it into the pot. Cover and steam the vegetables until they are just tender, which should take around 8 minutes. 4. Place the steamed vegetables on a serving platter and generously drizzle them with the Savory Goji Berry Cream. Finally, garnish the dish with chopped walnuts and sliced green onions.

Per Serving:
calories: 136 | fat: 9g | protein: 5g | carbs: 17g | fiber: 5g

Avocado Tartare

Prep time: 15 minutes | **Cook time:** 0 minutes | **Makes 2 cups**

¼ cup finely diced red onion
2 tablespoons capers, drained and minced
¼ cup minced fresh flat-leaf parsley, plus extra for garnish
1 teaspoon Dijon mustard
2 teaspoons fresh lemon juice
½ teaspoon gluten-free tamari soy sauce
1 teaspoon virgin olive oil (optional)
Salt and pepper, to taste (optional)
1 medium just-ripe avocado
4 to 5 drops of hot sauce (optional)
Crackers and crostini, for serving

1. In a medium bowl, mix together the diced red onion, capers, parsley, Dijon mustard, lemon juice, tamari, olive oil, and season with salt and pepper, if desired.
2. Cut the avocado in half, remove the pit, and gently peel the skin while preserving the flesh's integrity. Dice the avocado flesh into small pieces and add it to the medium bowl. Toss everything together to combine. If using hot sauce, add it and toss again. Taste the tartare and adjust seasoning as needed. 3. Garnish the avocado tartare with extra chopped parsley. Serve immediately with crackers or crostini. Enjoy!

Per Serving: (1 cup)
calories: 211 | fat: 18g | protein: 3g | carbs: 13g | fiber: 8g

Tandoori-Rubbed Portobellos with Cool Cilantro Sauce

Prep time: 25 minutes | **Cook time:** 10 minutes | **Serves 4**

Cool Cilantro Sauce:
½ cup raw sunflower seeds, soaked for at least 4 hours
¼ cup plus 2 tablespoons filtered water
1 clove garlic, finely grated
1 tablespoon fresh lime juice
1 tablespoon virgin olive oil (optional)
¼ cup finely chopped fresh cilantro leaves
1 green onion, white and light-green parts only, thinly sliced
Salt and pepper, to taste (optional)
Portobellos:
4 large portobello mushroom caps
2 tablespoons virgin olive oil (optional)
1 tablespoon fresh lime juice
1 tablespoon tandoori spice blend
1 (1-inch) piece of fresh ginger, peeled and finely grated
1 clove garlic, finely grated
Salt and pepper, to taste (optional)
Serve:
Warm cooked brown rice
Chopped fresh cilantro leaves

1. To prepare the Cool Cilantro Sauce, start by draining the sunflower seeds and transferring them to a blender. Add filtered water, garlic, lime juice, and olive oil (if using). Blend the mixture on high until you get a mostly smooth purée. If needed, scrape down the sides of the blender or add another tablespoon of water for the desired consistency. Transfer the sauce base to a small bowl and stir in the cilantro, green onions, salt, and pepper (if using). Cover the bowl and refrigerate the sauce until you're ready to use it. 2. Preheat your grill to high heat. 3. Next, prepare the Portobellos by taking the mushroom caps and using a spoon to scrape out the gills, which are the dark brown strips lining the underside of the mushroom. Place the scraped mushrooms on a plate. 4. In a medium bowl, whisk together olive oil, lime juice, tandoori spice, ginger, garlic, salt, and pepper. Rub this wet spice mixture on both sides of the portobello mushrooms. 5. Lightly oil the grill by rubbing it with a wad of paper towel. Place the spice-rubbed portobello caps on the grill and close the lid. Let them cook for 4 minutes, then flip them over and cook for another 4 minutes. The mushrooms should be tender, glistening lightly, and have char marks on both sides. Remove them from the grill. 6. Slice the grilled portobellos and serve them with the Cool Cilantro Sauce, warm rice, and garnish with extra chopped cilantro.

Per Serving:
calories: 261 | fat: 20g | protein: 6g | carbs: 18g | fiber: 3g

Baked Spaghetti Squash with Swiss Chard

Prep time: 15 minutes | **Cook time:** 55 minutes | **Serves 4**

2 small spaghetti squash (about 1 pound / 454 g each), halved
Salt and freshly ground black pepper, to taste
1 large bunch red-ribbed Swiss chard
1 medium yellow onion, peeled and diced small
1 red bell pepper, seeded and diced small
4 cloves garlic, peeled and minced
2 teaspoons ground cumin
2 teaspoons ground coriander
½ teaspoon paprika
½ teaspoon crushed red pepper flakes
Zest and juice of 1 lemon

1. Preheat the oven to 350°F (180°C). 2. Sprinkle salt and pepper on the cut sides of the squash. Place the squash halves, cut side down, on a rimmed baking sheet. Pour ½ cup of water into the pan and bake the squash for 45 to 55 minutes until it becomes very tender (a knife should easily pierce through the squash). 3. While the squash is baking, prepare the chard. Remove the stems from the chard and chop them. Chop the leaves into bite-size pieces and set them aside. In a large saucepan, sauté the onion, red pepper, and chard stems over medium heat for 5 minutes. Add water 1 to 2 tablespoons at a time to prevent sticking. Stir in the garlic, cumin, coriander, paprika, and crushed red pepper flakes, and cook for an additional 3 minutes. Add the chard leaves, lemon zest, and juice. Season with salt and pepper, and cook until the chard wilts, approximately 5 minutes. Remove from heat.
4. Once the squash is done baking, scoop out the flesh (which should resemble noodles) and mix it into the warm chard mixture.

Per Serving:
calories: 36 | fat: 0g | protein: 1g | carbs: 7g | fiber: 1g

Cumin-Citrus Roasted Carrots

Prep time: 10 minutes | Cook time: 30 minutes | Serves 6

8 large carrots, sliced into ½-inch rounds
¼ cup orange juice
¼ cup vegetable broth
1 teaspoon ground cumin
¼ teaspoon ground turmeric
Salt and black pepper (optional)
1 tablespoon fresh lime juice
Chopped flat-leaf parsley (optional)

1. Preheat the oven to 400ºF (205ºC). 2. Arrange the carrots in a large baking dish. Pour the orange juice and broth over the carrots, and sprinkle with cumin and turmeric. Season with salt and pepper, if desired. 3. Bake the carrots, uncovered, until they are lightly browned, and the liquids have reduced slightly, approximately 30 minutes. Remember to stir the carrots halfway through the baking process. Before serving, drizzle the carrots with lime juice and garnish with parsley, if desired. Enjoy!

Per Serving:
calories: 47 | fat: 0g | protein: 1g | carbs: 11g | fiber: 3g

Garlicky Winter Vegetable and White Bean Mash

Prep time: 20 minutes | Cook time: 25 minutes | Serves 4

Vegetable and Bean Mash:
2 cups peeled and diced celery root
2 cups chopped cauliflower
1 cup chopped parsnips
5 cloves garlic, peeled
1 cup cooked and drained white beans, such as navy or cannellini
¾ cup unsweetened almond milk
1 teaspoon virgin olive oil (optional)
Salt and pepper, to taste (optional)
Mushroom Miso Gravy:
1 tablespoon virgin olive oil (optional)
5 cups sliced mushrooms
2 teaspoons chopped fresh thyme leaves
4 cloves garlic, minced
Salt and pepper, to taste (optional)
2 teaspoons balsamic vinegar
1¼ cups vegetable stock
1 tablespoon mellow or light miso
2 teaspoons arrowroot powder
Freshly ground black pepper, for serving (optional)

Make the Vegetable and Bean Mash:
1. Place the diced celery root, cauliflower, parsnips, and garlic cloves in a medium saucepan. Cover the vegetables with cold water and place the pot over medium heat. Bring to a boil and simmer until the vegetables are tender, about 15 minutes. 2. Drain the vegetables and transfer them to the bowl of a food processor along with the white beans. Pulse the vegetables and beans a couple of times to lightly chop them. Add the almond milk, olive oil, salt, and pepper (if desired). Run the motor on high speed until you have a creamy and smooth mixture. Keep it warm.

Make the Mushroom Miso Gravy:
3. Heat the olive oil in a large sauté pan over medium heat. Add the mushrooms and let them sit for 2 full minutes. Stir them up and let them sear for another full minute. Add the thyme and garlic, and stir. After the mushrooms start to glisten slightly, season them with salt and pepper (if desired). Add the balsamic vinegar and stir. 4. In a small bowl, whisk together the vegetable stock, miso, and arrowroot powder until no lumps of miso remain. Pour this mixture into the pan with the mushrooms and stir. 5. Bring the gravy to a light simmer and cook until the gravy has thickened slightly. 6. Serve the Mushroom Miso Gravy piping hot on top of the vegetable mash. Sprinkle with freshly ground black pepper if you like.

Per Serving:
calories: 225 | fat: 6g | protein: 10g | carbs: 36g | fiber: 8g

Baked Spaghetti Squash with Spicy Lentil Sauce

Prep time: 15 minutes | Cook time: 55 minutes | Serves 4

2 small spaghetti squash (about 1 pound / 454 g each), halved
Salt and freshly ground black pepper, to taste
1 medium yellow onion, peeled and diced small
3 cloves garlic, peeled and minced
2 teaspoons crushed red pepper flakes, or to taste
¼ cup tomato paste
1 cup cooked green lentils
1 cup vegetable stock, or low-sodium vegetable broth, plus more as needed
Chopped parsley

1. Preheat the oven to 350ºF (180ºC). 2. Season the cut sides of the squash with salt and pepper. Place the squash halves, cut side down, on a baking sheet, and bake them for 45 to 55 minutes, or until the squash is very tender (it is done when it can be easily pierced with a knife). 3. While the squash bakes, place the onion in a large saucepan and sauté over medium heat for 5 minutes. Add water 1 to 2 tablespoons at a time to keep the onion from sticking to the pan. Add the garlic, crushed red pepper flakes, tomato paste, and ½ cup of water and cook for 5 minutes. Add the lentils to the pan and cook until heated through. Season with additional salt. Purée the lentil mixture using an immersion blender or in a blender with a tight-fitting lid, covered with a towel, until smooth and creamy. Add some of the vegetable stock, as needed, to make a creamy sauce. 4. To serve, scoop the flesh from the spaghetti squash (it should come away looking like noodles) and divide it among 4 plates. Top with some of the lentil sauce and garnish with the parsley.

Per Serving:
calories: 94 | fat: 0g | protein: 6g | carbs: 18g | fiber: 5g

Lemony Steamed Kale with Olives

Prep time: 10 minutes | Cook time: 20 minutes | Serves 4

1 bunch kale, leaves chopped and stems minced
½ cup celery leaves, roughly chopped
½ bunch flat-leaf parsley, stems and leaves roughly chopped
4 garlic cloves, chopped
2 tablespoons vegetable broth
¼ cup pitted Kalamata olives, chopped
Grated zest and juice of 1 lemon
Salt and pepper (optional)

1. In a steamer basket set over a medium saucepan, place the kale, celery leaves, parsley, and garlic. Cover and steam over medium-high heat for 15 minutes. Once done, remove from heat and squeeze out any excess moisture. 2. Set a large skillet over medium heat. Pour in the broth, then add the steamed kale mixture to the skillet. Stir frequently and cook for 5 minutes. 3. Take the skillet off the heat and add the olives and lemon zest and juice. Season with salt (if desired) and pepper, and serve. Enjoy!

Per Serving:
calories: 41 | fat: 1g | protein: 2g | carbs: 7g | fiber: 2g

Fermented Carrots with Turmeric and Ginger

Prep time: 15 minutes | Cook time: 0 minutes | Makes 8 cups

10 medium-large carrots, grated
½ medium cabbage, cored and thinly sliced with 1 leaf reserved
1 (3-inch) piece fresh turmeric, peeled and finely grated
1 (2-inch) piece fresh ginger, peeled and finely grated
1 small shallot, finely chopped
5 teaspoons fine sea salt (optional)

1. Combine the carrots, cabbage, turmeric, ginger, shallot, and salt, if using, in a large bowl and use clean hands to mix the vegetables together, squeezing and softening them until they are juicy and wilted. Transfer a handful of the mixture to a large widemouthed jar or a fermentation crock and press it down well with your fist. Repeat with the remaining carrot mixture, a handful at a time, and then add any liquid left in the bowl. The liquid should completely cover the mixture; if it does not, keep pressing the mixture down until it does. If they don't create enough liquid, add cooled brine to cover. You should have at least 3 inches of headspace above the vegetables. Clean the edges of the jar or crock of any stray pieces of vegetable. Place the reserved cabbage leaf on top of the vegetables. Add a weight, such as a small glass jar filled with water, a flat glass plate or lid, or a fermentation weight, to keep the vegetables submerged, then seal the jar or crock. Label and date it and put it in a cool, dark place for 10 days. 2. After 10 days, carefully remove the lid, as it might pop off because of the gases that have built up, then remove the weight and cabbage leaf and use a clean fork to remove a little of the carrots to taste. If the level of tanginess and complexity of flavor are to your liking, transfer the jar or crock to the fridge, or transfer the mixture to smaller jars and refrigerate. If not, replace the leaf and the weight, tighten the lid, set aside for a few more days, and taste again. Usually 2 to 3 weeks of fermentation results in a good flavor. The fermented carrots will keep in the fridge for months. The flavor will continue to develop, but at a much slower rate.

Per Serving: (1 cup)
calories: 37 | fat: 0g | protein: 1g | carbs: 9g | fiber: 3g

Baby Potatoes with Dill, Chives, and Garlic

Prep time: 5 minutes | Cook time: 20 minutes | Serves 2

2 cups water
12 baby potatoes
2 garlic cloves, minced
2 tablespoons chopped fresh dill
2 tablespoons chopped fresh chives
Pinch freshly ground black pepper (optional)

1. Combine the water and potatoes in a medium saucepan and bring to a boil over medium-high heat. Cook for 20 minutes or until the potatoes are soft when pierced with a fork. 2. Drain the liquid and add the garlic; then mix well. 3. Serve warm and top each portion with 1 tablespoon of dill, 1 tablespoon of chives, and pepper (if using).

Per Serving:
calories: 155 | fat: 1g | protein: 4g | carbs: 34g | fiber: 6g

Blackened Sprouts

Prep time: 10 minutes | Cook time: 20 minutes | Serves 4

1 pound (454 g) fresh Brussels sprouts, trimmed and halved
2 tablespoons avocado oil (optional)
Sea salt and ground black pepper, to taste
1 cup walnut halves
1 tablespoon pure maple syrup (optional)

1. Preheat oven to 425ºF (220ºC). Line a baking sheet with parchment paper, or grease it well. 2. In a medium bowl, toss the sprouts with the oil (if using). Season well with salt and pepper to taste. Arrange in a single layer on the prepared baking sheet. 3. Roast for 20 minutes, or until the edges start to blacken. 4. Meanwhile, place the walnuts in a bowl and drizzle with the maple syrup (if using). Toss until well coated. During the last 3 minutes of roasting time, place the coated walnuts on the same baking sheet as the sprouts to toast and caramelize. 5. Let cool slightly before serving.

Per Serving:
calories: 254 | fat: 20g | protein: 6g | carbs: 16g | fiber: 5g

Spicy Miso-Roasted Tomatoes and Eggplant

Prep time: 25 minutes | Cook time: 50 minutes | Serves 6

1 medium eggplant, cut into 1 x 3-inch wedges
4 medium tomatoes, cut into 6 wedges each
1 medium yellow onion, cut into ¼-inch slices
3 tablespoons melted extra-virgin coconut oil or olive oil (optional)
2 tablespoons unpasteurized sweet white miso
2 tablespoons mirin, or 1 teaspoon maple syrup (optional)
1 tablespoon freshly squeezed lemon juice
1 large garlic clove, grated or pressed
1 teaspoon ground coriander
1 teaspoon red chili pepper flakes
½ teaspoon ground turmeric
½ teaspoon fine sea salt, plus more to taste (optional)
¾ cup cooked chickpeas, well drained
Chopped fresh flat-leaf parsley or cilantro leaves for garnish

1. Preheat the oven to 400°F (205°C). 2. Line a large baking sheet with parchment paper and put the eggplant, tomatoes, and onion on it. Combine the oil, miso, mirin, lemon juice, garlic, coriander, red chili pepper flakes, turmeric, and salt, if using, in a small bowl and stir until smooth. Pour over the vegetables and toss until evenly coated. Spread the vegetables out on the pan; they should almost be in a single layer, with just a few overlapping. 3. Roast for 20 to 25 minutes, until the vegetables are browned on the bottom. Remove the vegetables from the oven and turn them over as best you can; you may end up just stirring them, as they will be juicy. Roast for another 15 to 20 minutes, until the vegetables are completely soft and browned in spots. Scatter the chickpeas over the vegetables, sprinkle with a little more salt, if using, and return to the oven for 5 more minutes to warm the chickpeas through. Transfer the vegetables to a serving platter and top with the herbs. Serve warm or at room temperature. Any leftovers can be stored in an airtight container in the fridge for up to 3 days.

Per Serving:
calories: 152 | fat: 8g | protein: 4g | carbs: 18g | fiber: 6g

Broccolini on Fire

Prep time: 5 minutes | Cook time: 20 minutes | Serves 2

1 bunch broccoli
2 tablespoons extra-virgin coconut oil (optional)
4 large garlic cloves, cut into ¼-inch slices
¼ teaspoon fine sea salt (optional)
½ teaspoon red chili pepper flakes

1. Trim the bottom ends of the broccolini stems. Cut the florets off the stems and further divide each floret into 2 or 3 pieces. Slice the stems in half lengthwise. 2. In a large heavy skillet, preferably cast iron, warm the oil over medium heat. Add the garlic and sauté for 4 to 5 minutes until it turns golden. Using a slotted spoon, remove the garlic from the pan, leaving the oil behind, and set it aside. Add the broccolini and stems to the pan and sauté for 12 to 15 minutes, stirring occasionally, until tender and lightly browned in parts. Remove from heat and stir in the salt (if desired) and red chili pepper flakes, along with the reserved garlic. 3. Serve the dish warm. Any leftovers can be stored in an airtight container in the fridge for up to 3 days.

Per Serving:
calories: 234 | fat: 14g | protein: 9g | carbs: 23g | fiber: 8g

Jicama-Citrus Pickle

Prep time: 15 minutes | Cook time: 0 minutes | Serves 6

1 small-medium jicama, peeled
2 tablespoons raw apple cider vinegar, or more to taste
1 teaspoon grated orange zest
1 teaspoon grated lime zest
1 teaspoon grated lemon zest
¼ cup freshly squeezed orange juice
2 teaspoons freshly squeezed lime juice
2 teaspoons freshly squeezed lemon juice
1¼ teaspoons fine sea salt, or more to taste (optional)

1. Slice the jicama into 1-inch pieces, and then use a mandoline or a sharp knife to cut it into thin slices lengthwise. Place the sliced jicama in a medium bowl, and add the vinegar, citrus zest and juice, and salt. Mix thoroughly to combine. Taste and adjust the vinegar or salt if needed. You can serve it immediately or store it in a jar in the refrigerator for up to 1 week. Enjoy!

Per Serving:
calories: 49 | fat: 0g | protein: 1g | carbs: 11g | fiber: 6g

Steamed Kabocha Squash with Nori and Scallions

Prep time: 10 minutes | Cook time: 15 minutes | Serves 4

½ medium kabocha squash with skin left on, seeded, and cut into wedges
1 sheet nori, toasted and crushed
2 scallions, thinly sliced, plus more for garnish
2 tablespoons tamari
1 tablespoon mirin
2 tablespoons raw unhulled sesame seeds, toasted

1. Set up a steamer and fill the pot with about 2 inches of filtered water. Bring to a boil over high heat and set the steamer basket in place. Arrange the kabocha wedges skin side down in the basket in a single layer and steam for 12 to 15 minutes, until the flesh is soft when pierced with a paring knife. 2. Meanwhile, combine the nori, scallions, tamari, and mirin in a small bowl; set aside. 3. When the squash is cooked, transfer to a serving platter and drizzle the nori mixture over the top. Sprinkle with the sesame seeds and scallions and serve. (Any leftovers can be stored in the fridge for 2 to 3 days.)

Per Serving:
calories: 37 | fat: 3g | protein: 2g | carbs: 7g | fiber: 1g

Roasted Balsamic Beets

Prep time: 5 minutes | Cook time: 50 minutes | Serves 6

6 medium beets, scrubbed
¼ cup plus 2 tablespoons balsamic vinegar, divided
2 teaspoons pure maple syrup (optional)
1½ tablespoons virgin olive oil (optional)
Salt and pepper, to taste (optional)

1. Preheat the oven to 400°F (205°C). 2. Trim both ends of the beets and peel them. Cut the beets into ½-inch dices. Arrange the diced beets in a single layer in a large glass baking dish. 3. Drizzle the diced beets with ¼ cup of the balsamic vinegar, the maple syrup, and the olive oil, if using. Season the beets with salt and pepper, if using, and gently toss them until they're evenly coated. Cover the dish with foil and place in the oven. 4. Roast the covered beets for 25 minutes. Then, remove them from the oven and add the remaining 2 tablespoons of the balsamic vinegar. Carefully toss the beets to coat. Roast the beets uncovered for another 25 minutes or until fork-tender. 5. Serve beets immediately or allow them to cool thoroughly on the counter. Beets can be stored in a sealed container in the refrigerator for up to 5 days.

Per Serving:
calories: 84 | fat: 4g | protein: 1g | carbs: 12g | fiber: 2g

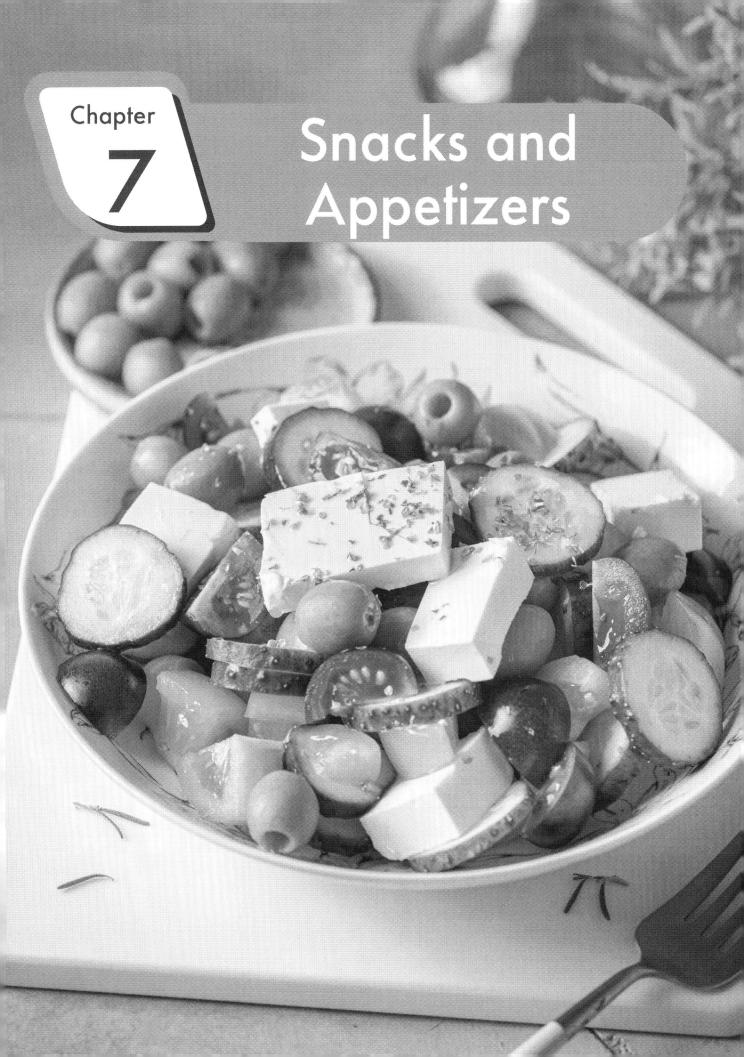

Chapter 7

Snacks and Appetizers

Protein Peanut Butter Balls

Prep time: 20 minutes | Cook time: 0 minutes | Makes 24 balls

- ½ cup creamy peanut butter
- ½ cup maple syrup (optional)
- ½ cup powdered soy milk, non-GMO
- ¼ cup flaxseed meal
- ½ cup coconut flour
- ¼ cup peanuts, chopped fine

1. In a medium bowl, combine the peanut butter and maple syrup (if using) thoroughly. Add the powdered soy milk, flaxseed meal, and coconut flour, and mix until well combined. Form the mixture into 24 balls. Lightly roll each ball in the chopped peanuts for coating. 2. Store the peanut butter balls in the refrigerator for up to 2 weeks. Enjoy these delicious treats whenever you like!

Per Serving: (2 balls)
calories: 133 | fat: 8g | protein: 10g | carbs: 12g | fiber: 2g

Slow Cooker Chipotle Tacos

Prep time: 15 minutes | Cook time: 4 hours | Serves 4

- 2 (15 ounces / 425 g) cans pinto beans, drained and rinsed
- 1 cup fresh, frozen, or canned corn
- 3 ounces (85 g) chipotle pepper in adobo sauce (about 2 peppers), chopped
- 6 ounces (170 g) tomato paste
- ¾ cup Thai sweet chili sauce
- 1 tablespoon unsweetened cocoa powder
- 1½ teaspoons taco seasoning
- 8 white corn taco shells or tortillas
- Favorite toppings:
- Spinach
- Lettuce
- Black olives
- Lime
- Avocado
- Peppers

1. Combine all the ingredients in the crockpot, except for the taco shells and toppings. Cook on low for 3 to 4 hours or on high for 1½ to 2 hours. 2. Once the filling is ready, generously spread it on your taco shells, whether they are hard or soft. Top them with your favorite toppings and enjoy a delicious taco feast.

Per Serving: (2 tacos)
calories: 484 | fat: 8g | protein: 20g | carbs: 65g | fiber: 19g

Savory Roasted Chickpeas

Prep time: 5 minutes | Cook time: 20 to 25 minutes | Makes 1 cup

- 1 (14-ounce / 397-g) can chickpeas, rinsed and drained, or 1½ cups cooked
- 2 tablespoons tamari or soy sauce
- 1 tablespoon nutritional yeast
- 1 teaspoon smoked paprika or regular paprika
- 1 teaspoon onion powder
- ½ teaspoon garlic powder

1. Set your oven to 400°F (205°C) and preheat it. 2. Mix the chickpeas with all the listed ingredients until well coated, then arrange them in a single layer on a baking sheet. 3. Bake for 20 to 25 minutes, remembering to toss them halfway through the cooking time to ensure they cook evenly.

Per Serving: (¼ cup)
calories: 106 | fat: 1g | protein: 6g | carbs: 17g | fiber: 5g

Orange Cranberry Power Cookies

Prep time: 10 minutes | Cook time: 10 minutes | Serves 12

- 1 cup dairy-free butter, softened
- 1 cup coconut sugar (optional)
- ⅓ cup orange juice
- 2 teaspoons organic vanilla extract
- 1½ cups whole wheat flour
- 2 tablespoons protein powder
- 1 teaspoon baking powder
- ¼ teaspoon baking soda
- 1 cup old-fashioned oats
- 1 cup dairy-free chocolate chips
- 1 cup chopped walnuts
- 1 cup dried cranberries

1. Preheat your oven to 375°F (190°C). 2. In the bowl of a stand mixer, cream together the butter and sugar (if using). Add the orange juice and vanilla extract, mixing well. 3. In a separate medium bowl, combine the flour, protein powder, baking powder, and baking soda. Add this dry mixture to the wet ingredients in the mixer, blending on medium speed until thoroughly combined. Then, stir in the oats, chocolate chips, walnuts, and cranberries on low speed. 4. Using heaping tablespoons of dough, drop the cookies about 2 inches apart onto an ungreased baking sheet. These cookies will be quite large and spread to 3 to 4 inches in diameter. Bake them for 10 to 11 minutes. 5. Allow the cookies to cool for a minute before transferring them to a wire rack to cool completely.

Per Serving: (2 cookies)
calories: 294 | fat: 21g | protein: 6g | carbs: 25g | fiber: 4g

Watermelon with Coconut-Lime Yogurt

Prep time: 10 minutes | Cook time: 0 minutes | Serves 1

- ¾ cup unsweetened coconut milk yogurt, plain or vanilla
- 1 teaspoon maple syrup (optional)
- Zest and juice of 1 lime, plus
- 1 lime cut into wedges for garnish
- 1¼ cups cubed seedless watermelon

1. In a small bowl, combine the yogurt with the optional maple syrup. 2. Zest one lime directly into the yogurt, then cut the lime in half and squeeze its juice into the mixture. Stir well to blend. 3. Serve the watermelon cubes alongside the coconut-lime yogurt. 4. Garnish the dish with lime wedges for added flavor. Enjoy!

Per Serving:
calories: 209 | fat: 3g | protein: 6g | carbs: 43g | fiber: 2g

Mango Plantain Nice Cream

Prep time: 10 minutes | Cook time: 0 minutes | Serves 4

2 plantains, peeled, cut into slices, and frozen
1 cup frozen mango pieces
½ cup unsweetened nondairy milk, plus more as needed
2 pitted dates or 1 tablespoon pure maple syrup
1 teaspoon vanilla extract
Juice of 1 lime

1. In a high-speed blender or food processor, blend together the frozen plantains, mango, milk, dates, vanilla, and lime juice for about 30 seconds. If needed, scrape down the sides and blend again until the mixture becomes smooth. If it appears lumpy, scrape down the sides once more and blend until desired consistency is achieved. Add more milk, 1 tablespoon at a time, if a smoother texture is desired.
2. For a smoothie-like consistency, refrigerate any leftovers in an airtight container. For a firmer ice cream texture, freeze the mixture. Before serving, allow the frozen treat to thaw slightly to achieve the desired serving texture.

Per Serving: (1 cup)
calories: 208 | fat: 1g | protein: 2g | carbs: 52g | fiber: 3g

Sunshine Everything Crackers

Prep time: 15 minutes | Cook time: 20 minutes | Makes 60 crackers

1 cup chickpea flour
1 cup certified gluten-free oat flour
2 teaspoons nutritional yeast
1 teaspoon fine sea salt (optional)
2 teaspoons garlic powder
1 teaspoon ground turmeric
Pinch of cayenne pepper (optional)
¼ cup plus 2 tablespoons coconut oil (optional)
¼ cup filtered water, plus extra if necessary
¼ cup mixed raw seeds

1. Preheat your oven to 350ºF (180ºC). 2. In the bowl of a food processor, combine chickpea flour, oat flour, nutritional yeast, sea salt, garlic powder, ground turmeric, cayenne pepper, and coconut oil (if using). Pulse the ingredients to lightly mix them, and then blend on high until you have a wet and uniform crumbly mixture. 3. While the food processor is on low, slowly pour the filtered water through the feed tube. The cracker dough should start forming a large ball. If it doesn't, add more water by the teaspoon through the feed tube until the ball forms. 4. Open the food processor lid and add the mixed seeds. Pulse the dough a couple of times to distribute the seeds. 5. Place a sheet of parchment paper, roughly the size of a large baking sheet, on the counter. Transfer the cracker dough onto the parchment and flatten it slightly with your hands. Cover the dough with another sheet of parchment paper. 6. Using a rolling pin, roll the cracker dough out to approximately ⅛ inch thickness, making sure it's even. Remove the top sheet of parchment paper. Carefully transfer the parchment with the rolled-out dough to a large baking sheet. Use a knife to score the dough into 1-inch square crackers. 7. Slide the baking sheet into the oven and bake until the edges of the crackers turn slightly brown, about 20 minutes. Allow the crackers to cool completely before storing them in a sealed container. They will stay fresh for about 5 days. Enjoy!

Per Serving: (6 crackers)
calories: 150 | fat: 9g | protein: 5g | carbs: 14g | fiber: 2g

Peanut Butter Chocolate Seed Balls

Prep time: 15 minutes | Cook time: 25 minutes | Serves 16

16 ounces (454 g) dairy-free chocolate chips
½ cup creamy peanut butter
½ cup raw shelled hempseed
½ cup unsweetened shredded coconut
1 cup sunflower seed kernels, pulsed fine in a mini food processor, divided

1. Melt the chocolate in a double boiler. Stir in the peanut butter and blend well. Take off of the the heat and mix in the hempseed, shredded coconut, and ½ cup sunflower seeds. Refrigerate until the dough is firm enough to use a small cookie scoop, about 30 minutes. 2. Remove the dough from the refrigerator and scoop out forty-eight balls. You can roll them into smoother balls with the palms of your hands. While they are still warm from rolling, roll them in the remaining pulsed sunflower seeds. 3. These will keep in the fridge for about 3 weeks and in the freezer for about 6 months.

Per Serving: (3 balls)
calories: 150 | fat: 9g | protein: 7g | carbs: 14g | fiber: 2g

Oat Crunch Apple Crisp

Prep time: 10 minutes | Cook time: 35 minutes | Serves 6

3 medium apples, cored and cut into ¼-inch pieces
¾ cup apple juice
1 teaspoon vanilla extract
1 teaspoon ground cinnamon, divided
2 cups rolled oats
¼ cup maple syrup (optional)

1. Preheat your oven to 375ºF (190ºC). 2. In a large bowl, toss the apple slices with apple juice, vanilla, and ½ teaspoon of cinnamon, ensuring all the apple slices are evenly coated. 3. Arrange the apple slices in the bottom of a round or square baking dish, and drizzle any remaining liquid over them. 4. In another large bowl, mix together the oats, maple syrup (if desired), and the remaining ½ teaspoon of cinnamon until the oats are fully coated. 5. Evenly spread the oat mixture over the apples, covering them entirely. 6. Bake for approximately 35 minutes, or until the oats take on a golden brown color. Serve and enjoy!

Per Serving:
calories: 213 | fat: 2g | protein: 4g | carbs: 47g | fiber: 6g

Sesame-Tamari Portable Rice Balls

Prep time: 20 minutes | **Cook time:** 25 minutes | **Makes 18 rice balls**

3 cups water
3 cups white sushi rice, rinsed
½ cup toasted white or black sesame seeds
2 tablespoons raw sugar (optional)
2 tablespoons reduced-sodium gluten-free tamari, or to taste
1 teaspoon ume plum or rice vinegar
1 tablespoon toasted sesame oil (optional)

1. Start by boiling water in a large saucepan. Once it's boiling, reduce the heat to medium-low, and add the rice. Stir frequently and let it cook for about 15 to 20 minutes until it becomes soft, moist, sticky, and tender, without being overly soggy.
2. After cooking, transfer the rice to a spacious bowl. Act swiftly and add all the sesame seeds except for 2 tablespoons, along with the sugar, tamari, and vinegar. Stir thoroughly to blend the flavors, allowing the mixture to cool slightly. 3. To prevent the rice from sticking to your hands, dampen them with water. Scoop about ½ cup of the rice mixture into your palms, gently but firmly pressing it to form a ball. Repeat the process with the remaining rice, and let the rice balls sit for 5 minutes.
4. Sprinkle the rice balls with the reserved 2 tablespoons of sesame seeds. Then, wrap them individually in plastic wrap or parchment paper. These rice balls can be refrigerated for up to a week or frozen individually for up to 3 months. When frozen, remember to thaw them overnight before enjoying.

Per Serving: (2 balls)
calories: 341 | fat: 6g | protein: 9g | carbs: 67g | fiber: 3g

Loaded Sweet Apple "Nachos"

Prep time: 5 minutes | **Cook time:** 0 minutes | **Serves 2**

3 apple, cored and cut into thin wedges
1 teaspoon ground cinnamon
2 tablespoons almond butter or tahini
2 tablespoons plain plant-based yogurt
1 tablespoon maple syrup (optional)
1 tablespoon raisins
2 tablespoons chopped nuts of choice
2 tablespoons unsweetened coconut flakes
1 tablespoon cacao nibs or vegan refined-sugar-free chocolate chips (optional)

1. Take a large plate and arrange the apple wedges in a single layer. Sprinkle the cinnamon evenly over the apples. Next, drizzle the almond butter, yogurt, and maple syrup over the apples. Lastly, sprinkle the raisins, nuts, coconut, and cacao nibs (if using) on top to complete the delicious treat. Enjoy!

Per Serving:
calories: 361 | fat: 15g | protein: 7g | carbs: 58g | fiber: 10g

Peanut Butter Snack Squares

Prep time: 10 minutes | **Cook time:** 20 minutes | **Serves 8**

½ cup coconut sugar (optional)
1 cup creamy peanut butter
1 teaspoon vanilla extract
¾ cup whole wheat flour
¼ cup garbanzo flour
1 teaspoon baking soda
½ teaspoon baking powder
1 cup old-fashioned oats
½ cup dairy-free milk
½ cup peanuts
½ cup dates, pitted and chopped small

1. Preheat the oven to 350°F (180°C) and lightly grease an 8-inch square baking dish.
2. Using a hand or stand mixer on medium speed, mix the sugar (if desired) and peanut butter for about 5 minutes. Add the vanilla and continue mixing. Gradually add the flours, baking soda, and baking powder, and mix on medium speed. Add the oats and briefly mix until the dough becomes stiff. Slowly pour in the milk and mix until just combined. 3. Fold in the peanuts and dates, ensuring they are well incorporated into the dough. 4. Gently press the dough into the prepared dish using your hands. Bake for 15 to 20 minutes or until the top is lightly golden brown.
5. Allow the baked bars to cool on a wire rack. Once cooled, cut them into sixteen squares and store in the refrigerator.

Per Serving: (2 squares)
calories: 366 | fat: 17g | protein: 14g | carbs: 44g | fiber: 7g

Mexikale Crisps

Prep time: 10 minutes | **Cook time:** 15 minutes | **Serves 2**

8 cups large kale leaves, chopped
2 tablespoons avocado oil (optional)
2 tablespoons nutritional yeast
1 teaspoon garlic powder
1 teaspoon ground cumin
½ teaspoon chili powder
1 teaspoon dried oregano
1 teaspoon dried cilantro
Salt and pepper to taste (optional)

1. Preheat your oven to 350°F (180°C) and line a baking tray with parchment paper. Set the tray aside. 2. Use paper towels to remove any excess water from the chopped kale leaves. Place the chopped leaves in a large bowl and add avocado oil, nutritional yeast, and seasonings. Mix and shake well, and add more nutritional yeast and additional seasonings if desired. Mix all the ingredients again to ensure even coating.
3. Spread the kale chips out on the prepared baking tray. Bake them in the oven for 10 to 15 minutes, checking every minute after the 10-minute mark until you achieve your preferred level of crispiness. Once done, remove the tray from the oven and let the kale chips cool down. 4. Serve and enjoy immediately, or store the kale chips in a container for later snacking!

Per Serving:
calories: 313 | fat: 14g | protein: 12g | carbs: 33g | fiber: 7g

Pump Up the Power Energy Balls

Prep time: 20 minutes | Cook time: 0 minutes | Makes 32 balls

- 1 cup old-fashioned oats
- ¾ cup almond meal
- ⅓ cup wheat germ
- ¼ cup flaxseed meal
- ¼ cup pepitas
- 2 tablespoons raw shelled hempseed
- 1 teaspoon ground cinnamon
- ¼ teaspoon ground nutmeg
- ½ cup dried currants
- ½ cup peanut butter
- ⅓ cup maple syrup (optional)
- 1 teaspoon vanilla extract
- ¼ teaspoon salt (optional)

1. In a medium bowl, combine the oats, almond meal, wheat germ, flaxseed meal, pepitas, hempseed, cinnamon, nutmeg, and currants. 2. In the bowl of a stand mixer, add the peanut butter, maple syrup, vanilla, and salt (if desired). Mix on medium speed until the wet ingredients are thoroughly combined. Pour the dry ingredients into the wet mixture and mix on low until everything is well combined. 3. Roll the mixture into thirty-two balls.

Per Serving: (3 balls)

calories: 168 | fat: 8g | protein: 10g | carbs: 22g | fiber: 4g

Baked Vegetable Chips

Prep time: 20 minutes | Cook time: 35 minutes | Serves 2

- 1 pound (454 g) starchy root vegetables, such as russet potato, sweet potato, rutabaga, parsnip, red or golden beet, or taro
- 1 pound (454 g) high-water vegetables, such as zucchini or summer squash
- Kosher salt, for absorbing moisture
- 1 teaspoon garlic powder
- 1 teaspoon paprika
- ½ teaspoon onion powder
- ½ teaspoon freshly ground black pepper
- 1 teaspoon avocado oil or other oil (optional)

1. Preheat your oven to 300ºF (150ºC) and line two baking sheets with parchment paper. Set them aside for later use. 2. Thoroughly scrub the root vegetables to remove any dirt, and make sure to wash and dry the high-water vegetables.
3. Using a mandoline or a sharp kitchen knife, slice all the vegetables into thin, ⅛-inch slices. Remember, the thinner the slices, the crispier the chips will be. 4. Lay the sliced high-water vegetables on a clean kitchen towel or paper towel. Sprinkle a generous amount of kosher salt over them, as this helps draw out excess moisture. This step is crucial for achieving crispiness. Let the vegetables sit for 15 minutes, then dab off any excess moisture and salt with a paper towel. 5. In a small bowl, combine garlic powder, paprika, onion powder, and pepper to create a flavorful spice mix.
6. Transfer all the vegetables to the prepared baking sheets, ensuring they form a single layer. Optionally, brush the vegetables with oil. 7. Evenly sprinkle the spice mix over the vegetables on the baking sheets. 8. Bake the chips for 15 minutes, then switch the pans between the oven racks for even cooking. Continue baking for an additional 20 minutes, or until the vegetables turn darker in color and develop crispy edges. 9. Once done, carefully transfer the chips to a wire rack to cool. The chips will become even crispier as they cool down, and you can enjoy their delicious crunchiness within a few minutes.

Per Serving:

calories: 250 | fat: 3g | protein: 8g | carbs: 51g | fiber: 6g

White Bean Caponata

Prep time: 10 minutes | Cook time: 0 minutes | Serves 4 to 6

- ¼ cup dry-packed, oil-free sun-dried tomatoes
- 1 (15-ounce / 425-g) can reduced-sodium white beans, drained and rinsed
- ½ cup unsweetened raisins
- ¼ cup grated carrot
- ¼ cup water-packed roasted red pepper
- ¼ cup green olives with pimentos
- 3 tablespoon red-wine vinegar
- 2 tablespoons pine nuts, toasted
- 2 tablespoons capers, drained

1. Place the sun-dried tomatoes in a small bowl and cover them with water. Allow them to soak for 5 to 7 minutes until they soften. Drain the tomatoes and chop them.
2. In a medium bowl, gently combine the sun-dried tomatoes, beans, raisins, carrot, roasted red pepper, olives, vinegar, pine nuts, and capers using a wooden spoon or spatula.

Per Serving:

calories: 182 | fat: 4g | protein: 8g | carbs: 32g | fiber: 7g

No-Bake Cereal Date Bars

Prep time: 15 minutes | Cook time: 15 minutes | Makes 16 bars

- 2 cups granola cereal
- 2 tablespoons flaxseed meal
- 2 tablespoons protein powder
- ½ cup chopped peanuts
- ½ cup dates, chopped small
- ½ cup almond butter
- ½ cup brown rice syrup
- ¼ cup maple syrup (optional)

1. Prepare an 8-inch square baking dish by lining it with parchment paper, leaving extra paper on opposite sides to act as handles for easy removal of the bars later.
2. In a large bowl, combine the cereal, flaxseed meal, protein powder, peanuts, and dates. 3. In a small saucepan, mix the almond butter, and both syrups, then bring them to a boil. Use a candy thermometer to cook the mixture until it reaches the hard ball stage at 260ºF (127ºC). Quickly pour the hot mixture into the cereal mixture and stir to combine. Spread the mixture into the prepared dish, using your fingertips to press it down evenly. Place the dish in the refrigerator for at least 30 minutes to cool.
4. Once chilled, grab the parchment paper "handles" and lift the bars out of the dish. Transfer them to a cutting board and slice into sixteen squares for serving.

Per Serving: (2 bars)

calories: 232 | fat: 13g | protein: 9g | carbs: 28g | fiber: 5g

Sweet Potato and Black Bean Quesadillas

Prep time: 10 minutes | Cook time: 20 minutes | Serves 4 to 6

Black Bean Spread:
1 (15-ounce / 425-g) can black beans, drained and rinsed
2 to 4 tablespoons chopped fresh cilantro stems and leaves
1 scallion, green and white parts, thinly sliced
1 tablespoon lime juice
1 teaspoon chipotle hot sauce
¼ teaspoon red miso paste
⅛ teaspoon garlic powder
Quesadillas:
1 pound (454 g) sweet potatoes, peeled and shredded
4 to 6 (8-inch) whole-grain tortillas
Hot sauce, for serving

Make the Black Bean Spread:
1. In a small bowl, use a fork to mash the beans until they reach a creamy texture.
2. Add in the cilantro, scallion, lime juice, hot sauce, miso, and garlic powder, and mix everything together.

Make the Quesadillas:
3. Heat a large nonstick skillet over medium heat. 4. Place the sweet potatoes in the skillet and cook, stirring occasionally, for about 10 minutes, until they are tender and lightly browned. Transfer them to a plate. 5. Wipe out the skillet and return it to the stove. 6. Divide the black bean spread (about ¼ cup to 6 tablespoons per tortilla) among the tortillas, spreading it evenly. 7. Divide the cooked sweet potatoes (about ¼ cup per tortilla) onto half of each tortilla, then fold the tortillas in half and press gently. 8. Place the filled tortillas in the hot skillet and cook for 2 to 5 minutes per side, until the tortillas become golden brown. 9. Remove the quesadillas from the heat and serve them with hot sauce.

Per Serving:
calories: 201 | fat: 1g | protein: 6g | carbs: 7g | fiber: 41g

Toast Points

Prep time: 5 minutes | Cook time: 20 minutes | Serves 2 to 4

8 whole-grain bread slices (thawed if frozen)
Balsamic vinegar, for brushing (optional)
Garlic powder, for seasoning

1. Place the bread in a single layer on a baking sheet lined with parchment paper.
2. Lightly brush the bread with vinegar (if using). 3. Sprinkle garlic powder over the bread. 4. Transfer the baking sheet to a cold oven, and then heat it to 350ºF (180ºC).
5. Once the oven reaches temperature, flip the bread over. Bake for an additional 5 to 15 minutes, or until the bread reaches your desired level of crispiness. Remove from the oven.

Per Serving:
calories: 165 | fat: 1g | protein: 8g | carbs: 31g | fiber: 6g

Cherry Chocolate Hemp Balls

Prep time: 20 minutes | Cook time: 0 minutes | Makes 24 balls

1 cup old-fashioned oats
½ cup unsweetened shredded coconut
½ cup chopped dried cherries
½ cup chopped pistachios
⅓ cup dairy-free chocolate chips
⅓ cup peanut butter
¼ cup maple syrup (optional)
¼ cup raw shelled hempseed

1. In a large bowl, combine all the ingredients thoroughly using a sturdy wooden spoon. Roll the mixture into 24 balls. 2. Store the balls in the refrigerator for up to 5 days, or freeze them for up to 6 months.

Per Serving: (2 balls)
calories: 1117 | fat: 6g | protein: 10g | carbs: 16g | fiber: 3g

Showtime Popcorn

Prep time: 5 minutes | Cook time: 1 minute | Serves 2

¼ cup popcorn kernels
1 tablespoon nutritional yeast
¼ teaspoon garlic powder
¼ teaspoon onion powder

1. Place the popcorn kernels in a paper lunch bag, folding over the top to prevent spills. 2. Microwave the bag on high for 2 to 3 minutes until there's a 2-second pause between popping sounds. 3. Take the bag out of the microwave and add nutritional yeast, garlic powder, and onion powder. Fold the top back over and shake to coat evenly. 4. Transfer the popcorn into a bowl and enjoy your tasty treat.

Per Serving:
calories: 48 | fat: 1g | protein: 4g | carbs: 6g | fiber: 2g

Garlic Hummus

Prep time: 10 minutes | Cook time: 0 minutes | Makes 3 cups

3 garlic cloves
2 (15-ounce / 425-g) cans chickpeas, drained and rinsed
3 tablespoons extra-virgin olive oil, plus more as needed (optional)
Juice of 2 lemons
¼ cup tahini
½ teaspoon salt
½ teaspoon ground cumin
1 tablespoon sesame seeds, for garnish (optional)

1. Place the garlic, chickpeas, olive oil, lemon juice, tahini, salt, and cumin in a blender. Blend the ingredients until you achieve a smooth and creamy texture. If you prefer a thinner consistency, you can add a bit more oil or water as needed.
2. Transfer the mixture into a serving bowl. For an extra touch, drizzle a little more olive oil on top and garnish with sesame seeds if desired. Enjoy!

Per Serving:
calories: 58 | fat: 4g | protein: 2g | carbs: 5g | fiber: 2g

Tortilla Chips

Prep time: 5 minutes | Cook time: 20 minutes | Serves 2 to 4

4 to 6 oil-free corn tortillas,
cut into triangles

1. Arrange the tortilla triangles in a single layer on a baking sheet lined with parchment paper. 2. Place the baking sheet with the tortillas in the cold oven, and then preheat the oven to 350ºF (180ºC). 3. Once the oven reaches the desired temperature, flip the tortilla triangles over. Bake for an additional 10 to 15 minutes, or until they become crispy.

Per Serving:
calories: 180 | fat: 3g | protein: 5g | carbs: 35g | fiber: 5g

Adventure Bars

Prep time: 5 minutes | Cook time: 0 minutes | Makes 8 bars

1 cup raw cashews
½ cup unsweetened shredded coconut
1 cup Medjool dates, pitted
½ cup dried apricots
½ cup dried tart cherries
4 tablespoons chia seeds
4 tablespoons hemp hearts
½ cup creamy almond butter

1. Using a food processor equipped with the chopping blade, pulse the cashews and coconut until finely chopped. Transfer the mixture to a bowl. 2. Add the dates to the food processor and pulse a few times before processing them into a paste. Incorporate the apricots and cherries with a few pulses. Return the cashew mixture to the fruit, and add the chia seeds, hemp hearts, and almond butter. Process until the ingredients form a cohesive mixture that holds together well when pressed. If the mixture appears too crumbly, add a little more almond butter or a splash of water, and process again. 3. Lay a piece of parchment paper on a clean, flat surface and transfer the mixture onto it. Press and shape the mixture into an 8-inch square that is slightly thicker than ¼ inch. Place it in the fridge or freezer to firm up before cutting into 8 bars. 4. Individually wrap the bars in parchment paper. They can be stored for several weeks in the fridge or several months in the freezer.

Per Serving:
calories: 322 | fat: 19g | protein: 8g | carbs: 34g | fiber: 6g

Peanut Butter Balls

Prep time: 0 minutes | Cook time: 30 minutes | Makes 12 balls

1 cup old-fashioned rolled oats
½ cup creamy peanut butter
¼ cup raisins

1. Combine all the ingredients in a large bowl, and use your hands to thoroughly mix them together. 2. Shape the mixture into small balls, each about the size of a tablespoon, using your hands. Place the balls on a baking sheet. 3. Freeze the baking sheet with the balls for 30 minutes. 4. After freezing, you can enjoy the treats immediately, or store them in an airtight container or plastic bag in the refrigerator for up to 5 days.

Per Serving: (2 balls)
calories: 168 | fat: 13g | protein: 8g | carbs: 14g | fiber: 4g

Apricot Pistachio Energy Squares

Prep time: 15 minutes | Cook time: 10 minutes | Makes 16 squares

1½ cups pitted dates, chopped
1 cup dried apricots, chopped
1 cup cashews, chopped
½ cup old-fashioned oats
½ cup pistachios
3 tablespoons cashew butter
2 tablespoons ground ginger
⅓ cup brown rice syrup
2 tablespoons maple syrup (optional)
1 teaspoon vanilla extract
¼ cup dairy-free chocolate chips (optional)

1. Line an 8-inch square baking dish with parchment paper and come up about 3 inches on opposite sides. This will act as a handle to remove the squares from the dish. 2. Add the dates, apricots, cashews, oats, and pistachios to a large bowl. Mix in the cashew butter and ground ginger and combine as well as you can. You can use your fingers to help blend it all together. 3. In a small saucepan, add the brown rice syrup, maple syrup (if desired), and vanilla. Bring to a boil and continue boiling until it reaches the hard ball stage, 260ºF (127ºC), on a candy thermometer. Quickly add to the date mixture and mix well. Pour into the prepared dish and press firmly and evenly into all edges and corners. Refrigerate at least 30 minutes. 4. Grab the "handles" of the parchment paper and lift out of the dish. Place on a cutting sheet and slice into sixteen squares. 5. If desired, melt the chocolate chips in a microwave or in a small saucepan. Drizzle back and forth over the bars.

Per Serving: (2 squares)
calories: 329 | fat: 14g | protein: 8g | carbs: 32g | fiber: 6g

Spicy Black Bean Dip

Prep time: 10 minutes | Cook time: 0 minutes | Makes about 2 cups

1 (14-ounce / 397-g) can black beans, drained and rinsed, or 1½ cups cooked
Zest and juice of 1 lime
1 tablespoon tamari or soy sauce
¼ cup water
¼ cup fresh cilantro, chopped
1 teaspoon ground cumin
Pinch cayenne pepper

1. In a food processor (preferably) or blender (if needed), combine the beans, lime zest, lime juice, tamari, and approximately ¼ cup of water. 2. Blend the ingredients until smooth, then incorporate the cilantro, cumin, and cayenne into the mixture.

Per Serving: (1 cup)
calories: 45 | fat: 0g | protein: 2g | carbs: 8g | fiber: 3g

Popeye Protein Balls

Prep time: 5 minutes | Cook time: 0 minutes | Makes 20 to 26 balls

1 cup raw hazelnuts	powder
¼ cup pumpkin seeds	1 teaspoon ground cinnamon
Handful of fresh baby spinach	Pinch of Himalayan pink salt (optional)
2 tablespoons raw cacao or carob powder	2 to 4 tablespoons superfood powder (açai, maqui, maca, spirulina, matcha or moringa), depending on potency, for dusting (optional)
1 cup raisins, soaked in water for 15 minutes, rinsed and drained	
2 tablespoons hemp protein	

1. In a food processor equipped with the S blade, combine all the ingredients except the superfood powder. Process the mixture until it forms a ball, taking care not to overprocess. Overprocessing may result in a softer dough. If the mixture becomes too soft, you can add up to 2 tablespoons of pumpkin seeds and refrigerate it for 30 minutes before shaping into balls. 2. To create the balls, use a tablespoon or your hands to scoop an appropriate amount of the mixture (as much as you like for one ball) and then roll it between your palms. 3. Place the formed balls on a plate and refrigerate them for at least 1 hour before serving. 4. If desired, before refrigerating, you can roll the balls in a plate of superfood powder to coat their exterior.

Per Serving:

calories: 167 | fat: 10g | protein: 5g | carbs: 15g | fiber: 2g

Slow Cooker Versatile Seitan Balls

Prep time: 15 minutes | Cook time: 6 hours | Makes 34 balls

1½ cups vital wheat gluten	¼ teaspoon ground ginger
½ cup chickpea flour	¼ teaspoon ground cloves
1 tablespoon mushroom powder	¼ teaspoon ground sage
½ teaspoon dried oregano	½ teaspoon salt (optional)
½ teaspoon onion powder	½ cup tomato sauce, divided
¼ teaspoon garlic powder	1 teaspoon liquid smoke
¼ teaspoon nutmeg	1½ cups vegetable broth, divided

1. In a large bowl, combine the gluten, flour, mushroom powder, oregano, onion powder, garlic powder, nutmeg, ginger, cloves, sage, and salt (if desired). Mix all the dry ingredients together thoroughly. 2. In a small bowl, mix together ¼ cup of tomato sauce, ¼ cup of water, liquid smoke, and ½ cup of vegetable broth until well combined. 3. Create a well in the center of the dry ingredients and pour in the tomato sauce mixture. Mix everything together until well incorporated, then start kneading the dough. Knead for about 1 minute until the dough becomes slightly elastic. It may be a bit sticky but should pull back slightly as you knead. 4. In a slow cooker, combine the remaining ¼ cup of tomato sauce, 1 cup of vegetable broth, and 3 cups of water, and stir to mix. 5. Tear off small chunks of the dough and shape them into round balls. You should have around forty-four balls. Alternatively, you can make seventeen larger balls and cut them after cooking and cooling, or create two logs and cut them into desired shapes. 6. Drop the dough balls into the liquid in the slow cooker. Cover and cook on low for 4 to 6 hours. The balls will increase in size as they cook. Check at the 4-hour mark to see if you like the texture; they will firm up further when refrigerated. 7. Remove the balls from the pot and let them cool. Store them in the refrigerator for up to 5 days or freeze them for up to 4 months. Enjoy as desired!

Per Serving: (½ cup)

calories: 161 | fat: 1g | protein: 30g | carbs: 10g | fiber: 2g

Skillet Cauliflower Bites

Prep time: 5 minutes | Cook time: 15 minutes | Serves 4 to 6

1 head cauliflower, cut into 1½- to 2-inch florets

1. Heat a nonstick skillet over medium heat and add the cauliflower. Cook, stirring every 3 to 5 minutes, for approximately 15 minutes, or until the cauliflower is browned and reaches a crisp-tender consistency. Remove from the heat.

Per Serving:

calories: 36 | fat: 0g | protein: 3g | carbs: 8g | fiber: 4g

Miso Nori Chips

Prep time: 10 minutes | Cook time: 15 minutes | Makes 48 chips

6 tablespoons almond or cashew butter	virgin coconut oil (optional)
¼ cup unpasteurized chickpea miso or sweet white miso	1 tablespoon filtered water
4 teaspoons mirin	8 sheets nori
1 tablespoon melted extra-	½ cup raw unhulled sesame seeds, toasted

1. Preheat the oven to 300ºF (150ºC). Line a rimmed baking sheet with parchment paper and set aside. 2. Combine the nut butter, miso, mirin, oil, and water in a small bowl and stir until smooth. Place one sheet of nori on a cutting board, top with 3 tablespoons of the miso mixture, and spread it evenly over the nori, all the way to the edges. Sprinkle with 2 tablespoons of the sesame seeds, top with another sheet of nori, and press to seal. Cut the stacked nori lengthwise in half and cut each half crosswise into 6 strips, to get 12 pieces. Arrange on the baking sheet and repeat with the remaining nori and miso mixture. 3. Bake for 10 to 15 minutes, until the nori is crinkled; the chips will crisp up as they cool. Remove from the oven and allow to cool. Store the chips in an airtight container for up to 2 weeks.

Per Serving: (2 chips)

calories: 50 | fat: 4g | protein: 1g | carbs: 3g | fiber: 1g

Chickpea Cookie Dough

Prep time: 20 minutes | Cook time: 0 minutes | Serves 8

1 (15-ounce /425-g) can chickpeas
½ cup smooth natural peanut butter
2 tablespoons pure maple syrup (optional)
1½ teaspoons vanilla extract
½ teaspoon ground cinnamon
2 tablespoons pecans

1. Pour the chickpeas into a bowl and fill the bowl with water. Gently rub the chickpeas between your hands until you feel the skins coming off. Add more water to the bowl and let the skins float to the surface. Using your hand, scoop out the skins. Drain some of the water and repeat this step once more to remove as many of the chickpea skins as possible. Drain to remove all the water. Set the chickpeas aside. Doing this gives the final product a smooth consistency. 2. In a food processor, combine the chickpeas, peanut butter, maple syrup (if using), vanilla, and cinnamon. Process for 2 minutes. Scrape down the sides and process for 2 minutes more, or until the dough is smooth and the ingredients are evenly distributed. 3. Add the pecans and pulse to combine but not fully process. 4. Refrigerate in an airtight container for up to 1 week.

Per Serving: (¼ cup)
calories: 170 | fat: 10g | protein: 6g | carbs: 15g | fiber: 3g

Peanut Butter Chocolate Bars

Prep time: 20 minutes | Cook time: 15 minutes | Makes 8 bars

1 cup peanut butter
10 pitted Medjool dates
1 cup instant oats
2 scoops organic pea protein
½ cup crushed dark chocolate
½ cup water
Optional Toppings:
Peanut butter

1. Preheat the oven to 257ºF (125ºC). 2. Add the oats, 5 Medjool dates and half of the water to a food processor and blend into a smooth mixture. Alternatively, add the ingredients to a medium bowl, cover it, and process using a handheld blender. 3. Line a loaf pan with parchment paper. Add the oats mixture to the loaf pan, spread it out and press it down firmly until it is 0.3 inch thick all over. 4. Add the pea protein, peanut butter, the remaining dates and water to a food processor and blend into a smooth mixture. Alternatively, add the ingredients to a medium bowl, cover it, and process using a handheld blender. 5. Add the peanut butter mixture in an even layer about 1-inch thick on top of the oats layer and press it down firmly to make it stick. 6. Transfer the loaf pan to the oven and let it bake for about 15 minutes. 7. Take the loaf pan out of the oven and add an even layer of the crushed dark chocolate on top. 8. Bake for another 10 minutes, take the loaf pan out of the oven, let it cool down and transfer to the fridge to let the mixture completely firm up for about 45 minutes. 9. Divide into 8 bars, serve cold with the optional peanut butter and enjoy! 10. Store the bars in an airtight container in the fridge, and consume within 6 days. Alternatively, store in the freezer for a maximum of 90 days and thaw at room temperature.

Per Serving:
calories: 374 | fat: 14g | protein: 17g | carbs: 23g | fiber: 14g

White Bean Tzatziki Dip

Prep time: 10 minutes | Cook time: 1 to 2 hours | Makes about 8 cups

4 (14½-ounce / 411-g) cans white beans, drained and rinsed
8 garlic cloves, minced
1 medium onion, coarsely chopped
¼ cup store-bought low-sodium vegetable broth, plus more as needed
Juice from one lemon, divided
2 teaspoons dried dill, divided
Salt (optional)
1 cucumber, peeled and finely diced

1. Place the beans, garlic, onion, broth, and half the lemon juice in a blender. Blend until creamy, about 1 minute, adding up to ¼ cup of additional broth as needed to make the mixture creamy. 2. Transfer the mixture to the slow cooker, stir in 1 teaspoon of dill, and season with salt (if using). Cover and cook on Low for 1 to 2 hours until heated through. 3. Meanwhile, in a medium bowl, mix the cucumber with the remaining 1 teaspoon of dill and the remaining half of the lemon juice. Toss to coat. Season with salt (if using). 4. Spoon the dip from the slow cooker into a serving bowl and top with the cucumber mixture before serving.

Per Serving:
calories: 59 | fat: 0g | protein: 3g | carbs: 11g | fiber: 4g

15-Minute French Fries

Prep time: 10 minutes | Cook time: 1 hour | Serves 6

2 pounds (907 g) medium white potatoes
1 to 2 tablespoons no-salt seasoning

1. Preheat the oven to 400ºF (205ºC). Line a baking sheet with parchment paper. 2. Wash and scrub the potatoes, then place them on the baking sheet and bake for 45 minutes, or until easily pierced with a fork. 3. Remove the potatoes from the oven, and allow to cool in the refrigerator for about 30 minutes, or until you're ready to make a batch of fries. 4. Preheat the oven to 425ºF (220ºC). Line a baking sheet with parchment paper. 5. Slice the cooled potatoes into the shape of wedges or fries, then toss them in a large bowl with the no-salt seasoning. 6. Spread the coated fries out in an even layer on the baking sheet. Bake for about 7 minutes, then remove from the oven, flip the fries over, and redistribute them in an even layer. Bake for another 8 minutes, or until the fries are crisp and golden brown, and serve.

Per Serving:
calories: 104 | fat: 0g | protein: 3g | carbs: 24g | fiber: 4g

Pressure Cooker Tender Patties

Prep time: 10 minutes | **Cook time:** 5 minutes | **Makes 2 cups**

¾ cup vital wheat gluten
¼ cup chickpea flour
2 tablespoons nutritional yeast
½ teaspoon dried basil
½ teaspoon salt (optional)
½ teaspoon poultry seasoning
¼ teaspoon garlic powder
¼ teaspoon onion powder
¼ teaspoon paprika
2¼ cups vegetable broth, divided
1 teaspoon extra virgin olive oil (optional)
½ teaspoon tamari
2 tablespoons tomato sauce

1. Add the gluten, flour, nutritional yeast, basil, salt (if desired), poultry seasoning, garlic and onion powders, and paprika to a large bowl. 2. Mix ¾ cup vegetable broth, oil (if desired), and tamari in a small bowl. Pour the wet mixture into the dry ingredients. 3. Mix and then knead for about 2 to 3 minutes or until elastic. It should be stretchy and pull back but still pliable. Divide the dough into eight pieces. Use your fingers to squeeze and work around into a patty measuring about 3 to 4 inches in diameter. 4. Place in an electric pressure cooker. 5. Add 1½ cups water, 1½ cups vegetable broth, and the tomato sauce to a small bowl, stir, and then pour over the seitan cutlets in the pressure cooker. Close the lid, making sure the top knob is turned to sealing. Press Manual on the front of the pot. Push button to 4 (meaning 4 minutes). In a few seconds, the pressure cooker will make a click and start to build pressure. It will take about 15 minutes to build pressure and cook. Leave the cutlets in the pot to set. They will cook more as the pressure is naturally releasing. Don't vent. 6. After about an hour, go ahead and vent. It may already have cooled completely, but vent to make sure all of the pressure has been released and then open the lid. 7. Remove the cutlets from the liquid and set aside to cool. You can eat them right away, add to a recipe, or keep in the fridge overnight. They are great the next day and keep well in the freezer.

Per Serving: (½ cup)
calories: 247 | fat: 2g | protein: 30g | carbs: 16g | fiber: 3g

Romesco-Style Hummus

Prep time: 10 minutes | **Cook time:** 0 minutes | **Makes 1½ cups**

1 teaspoon dry-packed, oil-free sun-dried tomato
1 (15-ounce / 425-g) can chickpeas, drained and rinsed
¼ cup water-packed roasted red pepper
3 tablespoons balsamic vinegar
2 tablespoons sliced or slivered almonds
¼ teaspoon garlic powder
¼ teaspoon onion powder
⅛ teaspoon smoked paprika

1. In a bowl, reconstitute the sun-dried tomato in water. Drain. 2. In a food processor, combine the sun-dried tomato, chickpeas, roasted red pepper, vinegar, almonds, garlic powder, onion powder, and paprika. Process until smooth and creamy.

Per Serving:
calories: 105 | fat: 2g | protein: 6g | carbs: 17g | fiber: 5g

Vanilla-Cinnamon Fruit Cocktail

Prep time: 10 minutes | **Cook time:** 0 minutes | **Serves 4 to 6**

1 pint blueberries
2 cups diced Granny Smith apples
1 cup halved mandarin orange slices
1 cup sliced strawberries
2 tablespoons lemon juice
2 tablespoons chia seeds
½ teaspoon vanilla extract
¼ teaspoon ground cinnamon

1. In a large bowl, using a wooden spoon or rubber spatula, mix together the blueberries, apples, orange slices, strawberries, lemon juice, chia seeds, vanilla, and cinnamon. Serve immediately, or refrigerate until serving.

Per Serving:
calories: 114 | fat: 2g | protein: 2g | carbs: 25g | fiber: 6g

Lemon-Pepper Bean Dip with Rosemary

Prep time: 10 minutes | **Cook time:** 0 minutes | **Serves 4 to 6**

1 (15-ounce / 425-g) can reduced-sodium white beans, drained and rinsed
1 tablespoon lemon juice
1 tablespoon red-wine vinegar
1 teaspoon freshly ground black pepper
½ teaspoon garlic powder
½ teaspoon dried rosemary
Pinch red pepper flakes

1. In a medium bowl, combine the beans, lemon juice, vinegar, pepper, garlic powder, rosemary, and red pepper flakes. Gently mix until combined (although this dip can be mixed and slightly mashed to create a chunkier texture).

Per Serving:
calories: 88 | fat: 0g | protein: 5g | carbs: 16g | fiber: 4g

Guacamole

Prep time: 10 minutes | **Cook time:** 0 minutes | **Makes 2 cups**

3 to 4 small avocados or 2 large avocados, diced
½ tablespoon lemon or lime juice
¼ cup finely diced red, white, or yellow onion
1 teaspoon minced garlic
¾ teaspoon ground cumin
2 tablespoons chopped cilantro
½ medium tomato, chopped
Pinch of salt (optional)
Freshly ground pepper, to taste

1. In a medium bowl, mash the avocados with a fork to the desired consistency. 2. Add the lemon (or lime) juice, onion, garlic, cumin, cilantro, tomato, salt (if desired), and pepper, and mix well.

Per Serving:
calories: 249 | fat: 22g | protein: 4g | carbs: 15g | fiber: 10g

Raw Date Chocolate Balls

Prep time: 20 minutes | Cook time: 0 minutes | Makes 24 balls

¾ cup sunflower seed kernels, ground
½ cup dates, pitted, chopped well
½ cup chopped walnuts
½ cup unsweetened cacao powder
½ cup maple syrup (optional)
½ cup creamy almond butter
½ cup old-fashioned oats (use gluten-free if desired)
¼ cup raw shelled hempseed
6 ounces (170 g) unsweetened coconut, for coating

1. Place the sunflower seeds, dates, walnuts, cacao powder, maple syrup (if desired), almond butter, oats, and hempseed in a large bowl. Mix well. 2. Pinch off pieces of dough and roll into twenty-four balls. Roll each ball in shredded coconut. Place in the refrigerator to harden for about 30 minutes.

Per Serving: (2 balls)
calories: 256 | fat: 16g | protein: 7g | carbs: 24g | fiber: 6g

Mocha Chocolate Brownie Bars

Prep time: 15 minutes | Cook time: 0 minutes | Serves 3

2½ cups chocolate or vanilla vegan protein powder
½ cup cocoa powder
½ cup old-fashioned or quick oats
1 teaspoon pure vanilla extract
¼ teaspoon nutmeg
2 tablespoons agave nectar (optional)
1 cup cold brewed coffee

1. Line a square baking dish with parchment paper and set it aside. 2. Mix the dry ingredients together in a large bowl. Slowly incorporate the agave nectar (if desired), vanilla extract, and cold coffee while stirring constantly until all the lumps in the mixture have disappeared. Pour the batter into the dish, while making sure to press it into the corners. Place the dish into the refrigerator until firm, or for about 4 hours. Alternatively use the freezer for just 1 hour. 3. Slice the chunk into 6 even squares, and enjoy, share, or store!

Per Serving:
calories: 213 | fat: 4g | protein: 27g | carbs: 17g | fiber: 4g

Nacho Cheese

Prep time: 5 minutes | Cook time: 10 minutes | Makes 3 cups

2 cups peeled and diced russet potatoes
1 cup sliced carrots
½ cup water
1 tablespoon lemon juice
½ cup nutritional yeast
1 teaspoon onion powder
1 teaspoon garlic powder
½ teaspoon salt (optional)

1. In a large pot, fill with water and add the potatoes and carrots. Bring to a boil over medium-high heat and cook for about 10 minutes, or until the vegetables are tender. Once done, remove from heat and drain the water. 2. Transfer the boiled potatoes and carrots to a blender. Add water, lemon juice, nutritional yeast, onion powder, garlic powder, and salt (if desired). Blend the ingredients until you achieve a smooth and creamy consistency.

Per Serving: (½ cup)
calories: 88 | fat: 1g | protein: 7g | carbs: 15g | fiber: 2g

Vanilla Almond Date Balls

Prep time: 20 minutes | Cook time: 0 minutes | Makes 20 balls

1½ cups almond flour
16 pitted dates
4 tablespoons sunflower seed kernels
4 tablespoons vanilla protein powder
2 tablespoons flaxseed meal
1 teaspoon vanilla extract
Pinch of salt (optional)
2 tablespoons sunflower seed kernels, ground fine in a small food processor

1. Place all the ingredients except the ground sunflower seeds in a food processor. Process on high until all is combined well and forms a ball. Transfer into a large bowl and form twenty balls. This dough works well by squeezing each one a few times to form a ball. Roll in ground sunflower seeds.

Per Serving: (2 balls)
calories: 131 | fat: 4g | protein: 8g | carbs: 23g | fiber: 4g

Nori Snack Rolls

Prep time: 5 minutes | Cook time: 8 to 10 minutes | Makes 4 rolls

2 tablespoons almond, cashew, peanut, or other nut butter
2 tablespoons tamari or soy sauce
4 standard nori sheets
1 mushroom, sliced
1 tablespoon pickled ginger
½ cup grated carrots

1. Preheat the oven to 350ºF (180ºC). 2. Mix together the nut butter and tamari until smooth and very thick. Lay out a nori sheet, rough side up, the long way. Spread a thin line of the tamari mixture on the far end of the nori sheet, from side to side. Lay the mushroom slices, ginger, and carrots in a line at the other end (the end closest to you). Fold the vegetables inside the nori, rolling toward the tahini mixture, which will seal the roll. 3. Repeat to make 4 rolls. 4. Put on a baking sheet and bake for 8 to 10 minutes, or until the rolls are slightly browned and crispy at the ends. Let the rolls cool for a few minutes, then slice each roll into 3 smaller pieces.

Per Serving: (1 roll)
calories: 62 | fat: 4g | protein: 2g | carbs: 3g | fiber: 1g

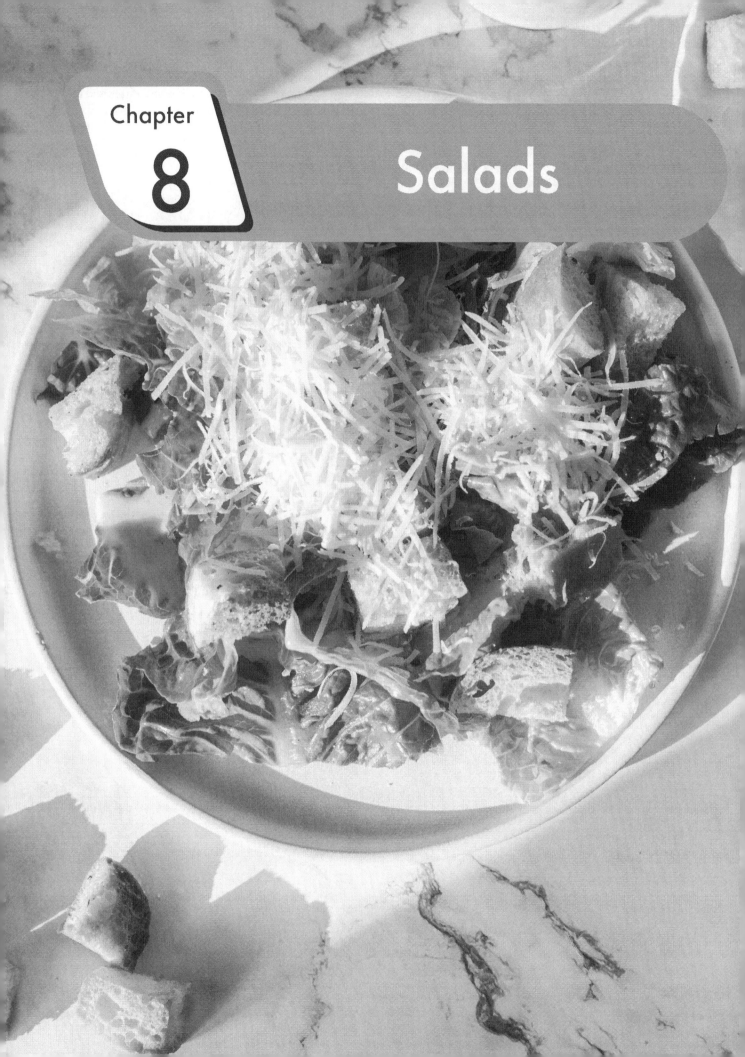

Chapter 8
Salads

Tuscan White Bean Salad

Prep time: 10 minutes | **Cook time:** 0 minutes | Serves 2

Dressing:
1 tablespoon olive oil (optional)
2 tablespoons balsamic vinegar
1 teaspoon minced fresh chives or scallions
1 garlic clove, pressed or minced
1 tablespoon fresh rosemary, chopped, or 1 teaspoon dried
1 tablespoon fresh oregano, chopped, or 1 teaspoon dried
Pinch sea salt (optional)
Salad:
1 (14-ounce / 397-g) can cannellini beans, drained and rinsed, or 1½ cups cooked
6 mushrooms, thinly sliced
1 zucchini, diced
2 carrots, diced
2 tablespoons fresh basil, chopped

1. Prepare the dressing by combining all the dressing ingredients in a large bowl and whisking them together. 2. Add all the salad ingredients to the dressing and toss them until well coated. For enhanced flavor, transfer the salad to a sealed container, shake it vigorously, and allow it to marinate for 15 to 30 minutes.

Per Serving:
calories: 146 | fat: 7g | protein: 4g | carbs: 17g | fiber: 5g

Kale, Black Bean and Quinoa Salad

Prep time: 20 minutes | **Cook time:** 30 minutes | Serves 6

2 garlic cloves, finely minced
½ yellow onion, diced
2 tablespoons water
2¼ cups no-sodium vegetable broth, divided
1 cup dried tricolor quinoa, rinsed
1 tablespoon freshly squeezed lemon juice
1 teaspoon lemon zest
1 teaspoon chia seeds
1 teaspoon smoked ancho chili powder
1 teaspoon ground cumin
6 cups chopped kale leaves
1 (15-ounce /425-g) can black beans, drained and rinsed
1 carrot, grated
1 red bell pepper, diced

1. In a large 8-quart pot over medium-high heat, sauté the garlic and onion with water for 2 to 3 minutes, until the water evaporates. Add 2 cups of vegetable broth and the quinoa. Bring it to a simmer, stirring occasionally, then reduce the heat to medium-low, cover the pot, and let it cook for 20 minutes. The quinoa is ready when it has a translucent center with a distinct ring around the edge and a chewy, not hard texture. Remove from heat and let it cool. 2. While the quinoa cooks, whisk together the remaining ¼ cup of vegetable broth, lemon juice, lemon zest, chia seeds, ancho chili powder, and cumin in a glass measuring cup. Let it sit for 5 minutes to thicken and let the chia seeds soak. 3. Place the kale in a large bowl and pour in half of the dressing, reserving the other half for serving. Use your hands to massage the kale and dressing together to soften the leaves. If you prefer even more tender kale, you can steam or blanch it before adding the dressing. 4. Stir in the quinoa, black beans, carrot, and bell pepper. Refrigerate for at least 1 hour before serving or, for best results, up to 1 day. Serve with the reserved dressing.

Per Serving:
calories: 207 | fat: 3g | protein: 10g | carbs: 37g | fiber: 10g

Cabbage Salad and Peanut Butter Vinaigrette

Prep time: 15 minutes | **Cook time:** 0 minutes | Serves 4

3 tablespoons creamy peanut butter
2 tablespoons rice vinegar
2 tablespoons full-fat coconut milk
1 tablespoon soy sauce
½ tablespoon maple syrup (optional)
2 cups shredded red cabbage
1 cup shredded green or red cabbage
1 cup chopped unsalted roasted peanuts

1. Whisk together the peanut butter, rice vinegar, coconut milk, soy sauce, and maple syrup (if using) in a medium bowl until well combined. 2. In a large bowl, combine the red and green cabbage along with the peanuts. Pour the dressing over the ingredients and stir thoroughly to coat everything evenly.

Per Serving:
calories: 329 | fat: 25g | protein: 14g | carbs: 17g | fiber: 5g

Mock Tuna Salad

Prep time: 10 minutes | **Cook time:** 0 minutes | Serves 4

Salad:
2 cups raw sunflower seeds, soaked in water for 2 hours
3 to 4 ribs celery, diced
2 scallions, diced
2 tablespoons dulse flakes
¼ cup fresh dill
Dressing:
⅔ cup hemp hearts
¼ cup coconut water or purified water
3 cloves garlic, peeled
½ cup fresh lemon juice
1 teaspoon sea salt (optional)
2 tablespoons stone-ground mustard

1. Begin by preparing the salad. In a food processor, pulse the sunflower seeds until they form a slightly chunky pâté. Transfer the sunflower seed pâté to a bowl. 2. Add the celery, scallions, dulse flakes, and dill to the sunflower seed pâté in the bowl. Mix all the ingredients together thoroughly and set the bowl aside. 3. Next, make the dressing. In a blender, combine all the dressing ingredients and blend until you achieve a smooth consistency. 4. Pour the dressing over the salad and toss everything together to ensure all the flavors are well combined. 5. Your delicious sunflower seed salad with a flavorful dressing is now ready to be served and enjoyed.

Per Serving:
calories: 403 | fat: 30g | protein: 13g | carbs: 19g | fiber: 9g

Mango Lentil Salad

Prep time: 10 minutes | **Cook time:** 0 minutes | Serves 2

- 2 cups cooked or canned red lentils
- 2 cups fresh or frozen mango cubes
- ½ cup fresh spinach
- 8 halved cherry tomatoes
- 2 teaspoons cumin seeds
- Optional Toppings:
- Shredded coconut
- Nigella seeds

1. If using dry lentils, soak and cook ⅔ cup of them as needed. 2. Blend the mango cubes and cumin together until smooth to make a purée. 3. Rinse the spinach thoroughly in a strainer and let it drain well. 4. Divide the spinach, tomatoes, and lentils into two bowls. Top each bowl with half of the mango purée and any optional toppings. Serve and enjoy! 5. Store the salad in an airtight container in the fridge and consume within 2 days. Alternatively, you can store it in the freezer for up to 30 days and thaw it at room temperature. The salad can be served cold.

Per Serving:
calories: 355 | fat: 1g | protein: 21g | carbs: 65g | fiber: 20g

Warm Sweet Potato and Brussels Sprout Salad

Prep time: 20 minutes | **Cook time:** 30 minutes | Serves 4

- 3 sweet potatoes, peeled and cut into ¼-inch dice
- 1 teaspoon dried thyme
- 1 teaspoon garlic powder
- ½ teaspoon onion powder
- 1 pound (454 g) Brussels sprouts
- 1 cup walnuts, chopped
- ¼ cup reduced-sugar dried cranberries
- 2 tablespoons balsamic vinegar
- Freshly ground black pepper, to taste

1. Preheat the oven to 450ºF (235ºC) and line a baking sheet with parchment paper.
2. Rinse the sweet potatoes in a colander and shake off excess water. Sprinkle the damp sweet potatoes with thyme, garlic powder, and onion powder, tossing them to coat evenly with the spices. Transfer the seasoned sweet potatoes to the prepared baking sheet, spreading them in a single layer. 3. Bake the sweet potatoes for 20 minutes, then flip them and continue baking for an additional 10 minutes or until they are fork-tender. 4. While the sweet potatoes roast, prepare the Brussels sprouts. Wash them and remove any tough or discolored outer leaves. Halve the Brussels sprouts lengthwise with a large chef's knife, then thinly slice the sprouts crosswise into shreds. Discard the root ends and loosen the shreds. 5. In a large bowl, combine the Brussels sprouts, roasted sweet potatoes, walnuts, and cranberries. Drizzle the mixture with vinegar and season with pepper to taste. Toss everything together until well combined. Serve and enjoy!

Per Serving:
calories: 360 | fat: 20g | protein: 10g | carbs: 44g | fiber: 12g

Succotash Salad

Prep time: 20 minutes | **Cook time:** 0 minutes | Serves 4

- 1½ cups cooked baby lima beans
- 3 ears corn, kernels removed (about 2 cups)
- 2 large tomatoes, chopped
- 1 medium red onion, peeled and diced
- ¼ cup balsamic vinegar, or to taste
- ¼ cup chopped parsley
- Salt and freshly ground black pepper, to taste

1. In a large bowl, mix all ingredient and mix well.

Per Serving:
calories: 221 | fat: 1g | protein: 9g | carbs: 47g | fiber: 9g

Green Mix Salad

Prep time: 10 minutes | **Cook time:** 0 minutes | Serves 2

- 1 head romaine lettuce, chopped
- 2 cups baby arugula
- 1 cup baby spinach
- 1 cup fresh cilantro, chopped
- 1 cup fresh parsley, chopped

1. Mix all the greens in a big salad bowl. Eat fresh or store in a closed container in the fridge for 2 to 3 days.

Per Serving:
calories: 74 | fat: 1g | protein: 5g | carbs: 13g | fiber: 8g

Quinoa Arugula Salad

Prep time: 10 minutes | **Cook time:** 20 minutes | Serves 4

- 1½ cups quinoa
- Zest and juice of 2 oranges
- Zest and juice of 1 lime
- ¼ cup brown rice vinegar
- 4 cups arugula
- 1 small red onion, peeled and thinly sliced
- 1 red bell pepper, seeded and cut into ½-inch cubes
- 2 tablespoons pine nuts, toasted
- Salt and freshly ground black pepper, to taste

1. Rinse the quinoa under cold water and drain. In a pot, bring 3 cups of water to a boil. Add the quinoa and bring the pot back to a boil over high heat. Then, reduce the heat to medium, cover the pot, and let it cook for 15 to 20 minutes, or until the quinoa becomes tender. Once cooked, drain any excess water and spread the quinoa on a baking sheet. Refrigerate it until it cools down. 2. While the quinoa is cooling, prepare the dressing. In a large bowl, combine the zest and juice of oranges and limes, along with brown rice vinegar, arugula, onion, red pepper, pine nuts, salt, and pepper. Once the quinoa has cooled, add it to the dressing mixture. Chill the quinoa salad in the refrigerator for 1 hour before serving. Enjoy the refreshing flavors!

Per Serving:
calories: 293 | fat: 6g | protein: 10g | carbs: 50g | fiber: 5g

Fava Bean Salad

Prep time: 25 minutes | Cook time: 0 minutes | Serves 4

- 4 cups cooked fava beans, or 2 (15-ounce / 425-g) cans, drained and rinsed
- 2 large tomatoes, chopped
- 4 green onions (white and green parts), sliced
- 1 large cucumber, peeled, halved, seeded, and diced
- ½ cup finely chopped cilantro
- 1 jalapeño pepper, minced (for less heat, remove the seeds)
- Zest of 1 lemon and juice of 2 lemons
- 2 cloves garlic, peeled and minced
- 1 teaspoon cumin seeds, toasted and ground
- Salt and freshly ground black pepper, to taste

1. In a large bowl, mix all ingredients and mix well. Chill for one hour before serving.

Per Serving:
calories: 152 | fat: 1g | protein: 11g | carbs: 31g | fiber: 12g

Warm Lentil Salad

Prep time: 10 minutes | Cook time: 15 minutes | Serves 2

- 2 teaspoons extra-virgin olive oil (optional)
- 2 garlic cloves, chopped
- 1 tablespoon Italian seasoning
- ½ head cauliflower, cut into florets (about 2 cups)
- 1 large carrot, peeled and diced small
- 2 medium tomatoes, diced small
- 10 Kalamata olives, pitted and halved
- 1 teaspoon salt (optional)
- ½ teaspoon black pepper
- 2 tablespoons balsamic vinegar
- 1(15-ounce / 425-g) can brown lentils
- 1 cup water
- 4 cups baby spinach
- 1 tablespoon sunflower seeds

1. Place a large saucepan on the stove over medium heat and add the olive oil. Once the oil is heated, add the minced garlic and Italian seasoning. Sauté for 2 to 3 minutes until the aroma of the herbs and garlic fills the air. 2. Introduce the cauliflower, carrot, tomatoes, olives, and season with salt (if using) and black pepper. Stir frequently and cook for another 2 to 3 minutes, allowing the flavors to meld together. Pour in the balsamic vinegar, and cook for an additional 2 to 3 minutes to let the sugars caramelize slightly. 3. Incorporate the lentils and water into the mixture. Bring it to a boil, and let it simmer for 2 to 3 minutes until everything is heated through and well-combined. Remove the saucepan from the heat. 4. In a spacious bowl, combine the fresh spinach and sunflower seeds. Add the lentil mixture to the bowl and toss until the spinach starts to wilt slightly, blending all the ingredients together. Enjoy your hearty and nutritious lentil salad!

Per Serving:
calories: 363 | fat: 10g | protein: 21g | carbs: 53g | fiber: 19g

Strawberry-Pistachio Salad

Prep time: 10 minutes | Cook time: 0 minutes | Serves 6

- ¼ cup orange juice
- 2 tablespoons fresh lime juice
- ¼ teaspoon salt, plus more to taste (optional)
- ⅛ teaspoon black pepper, plus more to taste
- ½ small red onion, chopped or sliced
- 2 cups cooked grains, cooled
- 2 cups strawberries, hulled and chopped
- 1½ cups cooked cannellini beans, drained and rinsed
- 1 (5 to 6 ounces / 142 to 170 g) container mixed baby greens
- ½ cup chopped cilantro
- ½ cup roasted, shelled pistachios, chopped
- ½ avocado, diced
- High-quality balsamic vinegar

1. In a large bowl, mix together the orange juice, lime juice, ¼ teaspoon salt (if desired), and ⅛ teaspoon pepper to create the dressing. Add the onions to the dressing and toss them until coated. Then, add the grains, strawberries, and beans, and gently toss to combine all the ingredients. 2. Taste the salad and adjust the seasoning with salt and pepper according to your preference. If not serving immediately, cover the bowl and refrigerate the salad for up to 1 day. 3. Just before serving, add the greens and cilantro to the salad and toss to combine everything. Sprinkle the pistachios over the top, add the avocado slices for extra richness, and drizzle with vinegar for added tanginess. Serve and enjoy this vibrant and flavorful salad!

Per Serving:
calories: 393 | fat: 10g | protein: 11g | carbs: 67g | fiber: 8g

Tomato, Corn and Bean Salad

Prep time: 20 minutes | Cook time: 10 minutes | Serves 4

- 6 ears corn
- 3 large tomatoes, diced
- 2 cups cooked navy beans, or 1 (15-ounce / 425-g) can, drained and rinsed
- 1 medium red onion, peeled and diced small
- 1 cup finely chopped basil
- 2 tablespoons balsamic vinegar
- Salt and freshly ground black pepper, to taste

1. Fill a large pot with water and bring it to a rolling boil. Add the corn and cook for 7 to 10 minutes until tender. Drain the water from the pot and immediately rinse the corn under cold water to cool it down. Once cooled, carefully cut the kernels from the cob. 2. In a spacious bowl, combine the fresh corn kernels, tomatoes, beans, onion, basil, balsamic vinegar, and season with salt and pepper. Toss all the ingredients together until they are well mixed. Chill the salad in the refrigerator for 1 hour before serving to let the flavors meld and enjoy a refreshing and delightful summer dish.

Per Serving:
calories: 351 | fat: 2g | protein: 15g | carbs: 66g | fiber: 17g

Spinach Salad with Sweet Smoky Dressing

Prep time: 15 minutes | Cook time: 0 minutes | Serves 4 to 6

Dressing:
¼ cup balsamic vinegar
2 tablespoons soy sauce
3 tablespoons pure maple syrup
1½ tablespoons Dijon mustard
½ teaspoon smoked paprika
Salad:
4 to 6 cups spinach
2 cups sliced strawberries
¼ red or white onion, thinly sliced and rinsed

Preparing the Dressing:
1. In a small bowl or a container with a lid, whisk together the vinegar, soy sauce, maple syrup, mustard, and paprika until well combined. Alternatively, if using a container with a lid, you can shake the ingredients together.

Creating the Salad:
2. In a large bowl, combine the fresh spinach, strawberries, and onion.

Bringing it Together:
3. Pour the dressing over the salad and toss everything together until the ingredients are coated with the dressing. Serve immediately and enjoy your delicious and refreshing salad!

Per Serving:
calories: 84 | fat: 1g | protein: 2g | carbs: 18g | fiber: 3g

Apple Broccoli Crunch Bowl

Prep time: 20 minutes | Cook time: 0 minutes | Serves 6

Bowl:
2 medium heads broccoli
3 diced apples
¼ cup diced red onion
½ cup raisins
½ cup sunflower seed kernels
¼ cup raw shelled hempseed
Dressing:
¼ cup cider vinegar
½ cup extra virgin olive oil (optional)
2 cloves garlic, minced
1 tablespoon maple syrup (optional)
½ teaspoon salt (optional)
¼ teaspoon ground black pepper

Prepare the Bowl:
1. Start by cutting the broccoli florets from the stalks and set the stalks aside. Take the florets and chop them into very small pieces. Place the chopped florets in a spacious bowl. 2. Now, remove the tough outer skin from the broccoli stalks to reveal the tender inside. Discard the outer skin. Slice the inner stalks into matchstick-sized pieces. Alternatively, you can use a mandolin or a food processor with an appropriate attachment to achieve long strips of broccoli stems (not grated). Another option is to use scissors to cut the stems into small sticks that will retain their shape. Add these prepared stems to the same large bowl along with the florets. Also, include the diced apples, onions, raisins, sunflower seeds, and hempseed.

Make the Dressing:
3. In a separate medium bowl, whisk together all the dressing ingredients until well combined. This will create a flavorful dressing with a harmonious blend of tastes. Pour the dressing over the salad in the large bowl and toss everything together, ensuring that the dressing coats all the ingredients evenly. Chill until Ready to Serve:
4. Once the salad is dressed, let it chill in the refrigerator until you're ready to serve. This chilling period allows the flavors to meld, creating a delightful and refreshing dish. Enjoy your delicious and nutritious broccoli salad when it's time to serve!

Per Serving:
calories: 296 | fat: 24g | protein: 9g | carbs: 18g | fiber: 4g

Lentil, Lemon and Mushroom Salad

Prep time: 10 minutes | Cook time: 25 minutes | Serves 2

½ cup dry lentils of choice
2 cups vegetable broth
3 cups mushrooms, thickly sliced
1 cup sweet or purple onion, chopped
4 teaspoons extra virgin olive oil (optional)
2 tablespoons garlic powder or
3 garlic cloves, minced
¼ teaspoon chili flakes
1 tablespoon lemon juice
2 tablespoons cilantro, chopped
½ cup arugula
Salt and pepper to taste (optional)

To sprout the lentils, follow these steps for 2 to 3 days:
1. Rinse the lentils thoroughly under cold water and drain them.
2. Place the lentils in a sprouting jar or a fine-mesh sieve. Cover with a clean cloth and secure with a rubber band.
3. Rinse the lentils with fresh water 2 to 3 times a day, ensuring they stay moist.
4. After 2 to 3 days, you'll have sprouted lentils ready to use.

For the Mushroom and Lentil Salad:
1. In a deep saucepan, bring vegetable stock to a boil. Add the sprouted lentils and cook for about 5 minutes over low heat until they are slightly tender. Remove from heat, drain the excess water, and set aside. 2. In a frying pan over high heat, add 2 tablespoons of olive oil. Stir in the onions, garlic, and chili flakes, cooking until the onions are almost translucent (about 5 to 10 minutes), stirring frequently. Add the mushrooms to the pan and continue cooking until the onions are completely translucent, and the mushrooms have softened. Remove the pan from heat.
3. In a large bowl, mix the cooked lentils, onions, mushrooms, and garlic. Add the lemon juice and the remaining olive oil, tossing or stirring until all the ingredients are thoroughly combined. 4. To serve, place the mushroom and lentil mixture over a bed of arugula in a bowl. Season with salt and pepper to taste, if desired. Alternatively, you can store the salad for later enjoyment.

Per Serving:
calories: 262 | fat: 10g | protein: 16g | carbs: 28g | fiber: 15g

Vegan "Toona" Salad

Prep time: 10 minutes | Cook time: 0 minutes | Serves 4

3 cups cooked chickpeas
1 avocado, peeled and pitted
½ cup chopped red onion
¼ cup chopped celery
2 tablespoons Dijon mustard
1½ tablespoons freshly squeezed lemon juice
½ tablespoon maple syrup (optional)
1 teaspoon garlic powder

1. In a large bowl, combine the chickpeas and the avocado. Using a fork or a potato masher, smash them down until the majority of the chickpeas have been broken apart. 2. Stir in the onion, celery, mustard, lemon juice, maple syrup (if desired), and garlic powder, making sure everything is thoroughly combined, and serve.

Per Serving:
calories: 298 | fat: 10g | protein: 13g | carbs: 42g | fiber: 13g

Broccoli Caesar with Smoky Tempeh Bits

Prep time: 20 minutes | Cook time: 10 minutes | Serves 4

Creamy Cashew Caesar Dressing:
2 tablespoons raw cashew butter
2 tablespoons filtered water
1½ tablespoons fresh lemon juice
salt and pepper, to taste (optional)
3 cloves garlic, grated
1 teaspoon Dijon mustard
1 teaspoon minced capers
1 tablespoon nutritional yeast
3 tablespoons virgin olive oil (optional)
Salad:
Pinch of salt (optional)
1 bunch broccoli, cut into florets
1 teaspoon sweet paprika
1 teaspoon smoked paprika
1 teaspoon pure maple syrup (optional)
1 teaspoon apple cider vinegar
½ teaspoon gluten-free tamari soy sauce
2 teaspoons virgin olive oil (optional)
½ block (4 ounces / 113 g) tempeh, crumbled
Garnishes:
2 teaspoons nutritional yeast
Freshly ground black pepper

1. Make the Creamy Cashew Caesar Dressing: In a jar with a tight-fitting lid, combine the cashew butter, water, lemon juice, salt, and pepper, if using. Stir this mixture with a spoon or small spatula until the cashew butter is broken up. Mash the chunks of cashew butter against the sides of the jar to get it as integrated as possible. Add the garlic, Dijon mustard, capers, nutritional yeast, and olive oil, if using. Tightly secure the lid, and shake the jar vigorously until the dressing has a smooth and creamy consistency. Set aside. 2. Make the Salad: Bring a large saucepan of water to a boil over medium-high heat. Add a fat pinch of salt and the broccoli florets, and simmer until the broccoli is just tender and bright green, about 4 minutes. Drain the broccoli and run under cold water to stop the cooking process. Set aside. 3. In a small bowl, stir together the paprika, smoked paprika, maple syrup, if using, apple cider vinegar, and tamari. Set aside. 4. Dry the saucepan and return it to the stove over medium heat. Add the oil and let it heat through until it's shimmering slightly. Add the crumbled tempeh, spreading it out to a single layer. Let it sit and brown for a full 2 minutes. Then stir it up, and let it sit another full minute. Pour the paprika mixture into the pan. It should sizzle quite a bit. Stir it to coat all of the tempeh. Remove from the heat. 5. Place the broccoli on your serving platter. Drizzle the Creamy Cashew Caesar Dressing over the top. Scatter the smoky tempeh bits over the top as well. Garnish with some nutritional yeast and freshly ground black pepper to finish. Serve immediately.

Per Serving:
calories: 204 | fat: 19g | protein: 9g | carbs: 10g | fiber: 2g

Greek Salad in a Jar

Prep time: 10 minutes | Cook time: 10 minutes | Serves 4

Salad:
1 cup uncooked quinoa
1 cucumber, diced
2 cups cherry tomatoes, halved
2 bell peppers, seeded and chopped
½ cup walnuts, chopped
¼ cup sun-dried black olives, sliced
4 cups chopped mixed greens (romaine is great, too)
Dressing:
¼ cup extra-virgin olive oil
(optional)
½ cup fresh lemon juice
1 tablespoon Dijon mustard
3 cloves garlic, minced, or 2 teaspoons garlic powder
¼ cup basil, finely chopped, or 1 tablespoon dried
1 tablespoon chopped fresh oregano, or 1 teaspoon dried
Himalayan pink salt and freshly ground black pepper (about ¼ teaspoon each)

Creating the Salad:
1. Cook the quinoa according to the package directions and set it aside to cool.
Preparing the Dressing:
2. In a small jar or a container with a lid, combine all the dressing ingredients. Secure the lid tightly and shake the jar to thoroughly blend the dressing.
Assembling the Salad:
3. Start by adding 1 to 4 tablespoons of dressing to the bottom of each jar, adjusting the amount to your taste. 4. Layer the ingredients in the following order: cucumber, cooked quinoa, tomatoes, bell peppers, walnuts, and olives. Finally, top it off with the chopped mixed greens to fill the jar.
Storing the Salad:
5. Securely screw the lid on each jar and store the salads in the refrigerator. They will remain fresh and delicious for up to 4 days.
Enjoying the Salad:
6. When you're ready to eat, unscrew the lid and pour the salad into a bowl. As you do so, the dressing will coat the ingredients. If needed, gently toss the salad with a fork to ensure everything is well combined. Now you have a convenient and delightful salad ready to enjoy whenever you please!

Per Serving:
calories: 399 | fat: 24g | protein: 10g | carbs: 39g | fiber: 6g

Provencal Beans and Tomato Salad

Prep time: 10 minutes | Cook time: 0 minutes | Serves 2

2 cups cooked or canned white beans
1 small red onion, minced
8 halved cherry tomatoes
¼ cup lemon juice
3 tablespoons dried Provencal herbs

Optional Toppings:
Pine nuts
Black pepper

1. When using dry white beans, soak and cook ⅔ cup of dry white beans if necessary. 2. Transfer the white beans to a large bowl, and add the minced red onion, halved cherry tomatoes, lemon juice and herbs. 3. Stir thoroughly using a spatula and make sure everything is mixed evenly. 4. Divide the white beans salad between two bowls, garnish with the optional toppings, serve and enjoy! 5. Store the salad in an airtight container in the fridge, and consume within 2 days. Alternatively, store in the freezer for a maximum of 30 days and thaw at room temperature. The salad can be served cold.

Per Serving:
calories: 311 | fat: 1g | protein: 20g | carbs: 56g | fiber: 14g

Forbidden Black Rice and Edamame Salad

Prep time: 10 minutes | Cook time: 30 minutes | Serves 4

Salad:
1 cup black rice
2 cups water
Pinch sea salt (optional)
1 large sweet potato
1 teaspoon olive oil (optional)
1 cup shelled frozen edamame, thawed
1 red bell pepper, seeded and chopped
½ head broccoli, chopped
4 scallions, chopped
Fresh cilantro, chopped
Sesame seeds

Dressing:
Juice of ½ orange, or ½ cup pure orange juice
1 tablespoon soy sauce
1 tablespoon rice vinegar or apple cider vinegar
2 teaspoons maple syrup (optional)
2 teaspoons sesame oil (optional)

1. Preheat your oven to 400ºF (205ºC). 2. In a medium pot, combine the rice, water, and optional salt. Bring it to a boil over high heat, then cover and let it simmer for about 30 minutes until the rice becomes soft. 3. While the rice is cooking, peel and dice the sweet potato into small cubes. If you prefer, toss the cubes with olive oil. Spread the sweet potato cubes on a 9-inch square baking dish and roast them in the preheated oven for 15 to 20 minutes until they turn tender. 4. As the rice and sweet potato cubes cool, make the dressing. In a jar, combine all the dressing ingredients, then give it a good shake to blend everything well. 5. In a large bowl, mix the cooked rice, roasted sweet potato cubes, edamame, bell pepper, broccoli, and scallions. Pour the dressing over the salad and toss to coat all the ingredients. Sprinkle some chopped fresh cilantro and sesame seeds on top for added flavor and presentation.

Per Serving:
calories: 224 | fat: 11g | protein: 9g | carbs: 30g | fiber: 10g

Bulgur, Cucumber and Tomato Salad

Prep time: 15 minutes | Cook time: 10 minutes | Serves 4

1½ cups bulgur
1 cup cherry tomatoes, halved
1 medium cucumber, halved, seeded, and diced
3 cloves garlic, peeled and minced
4 green onions (white and green parts), sliced
Zest and juice of 2 lemons
2 tablespoons red wine vinegar
1 teaspoon crushed red pepper flakes, or to taste
¼ cup minced tarragon
Salt and freshly ground black pepper, to taste

1. Bring 3 cups of water to a boil in a medium pot and add the bulgur. Remove the pot from the heat, cover with a tight-fitting lid, and let it sit until the water is absorbed and the bulgur is tender, about 15 minutes. Spread the bulgur on a baking sheet and let cool to room temperature. 2. Transfer the cooled bulgur to a bowl, add all the remaining ingredients, and mix well to combine. Chill for 1 hour before serving.

Per Serving:
calories: 207 | fat: 0g | protein: 7g | carbs: 45g | fiber: 8g

White Beans Summer Salad

Prep time: 10 minutes | Cook time: 0 minutes | Serves 2

2 cups cooked or canned white beans
½ cubed cucumber
8 sun-dried tomatoes, minced
4 tangerines
1 tablespoon fresh or dried thyme

Optional Toppings:
Black pepper
Tahini

1. When using dry white beans, soak and cook ⅔ cup of dry white beans if necessary. 2. Transfer the white beans to a large bowl, and add the minced sun-dried tomatoes, cucumber cubes and thyme. If using fresh thyme, chop it finely before adding it to the bowl. 3. Stir thoroughly using a spatula and make sure everything is mixed evenly. 4. Peel and section the tangerines and set them aside to garnish the salad. 5. Divide the white beans salad between two bowls, garnish with the tangerine and the optional toppings, serve and enjoy! 6. Store the salad in an airtight container in the fridge, and consume within 2 days. Alternatively, store in the freezer for a maximum of 30 days and thaw at room temperature. The salad can be served cold.

Per Serving:
calories: 376 | fat: 2g | protein: 22g | carbs: 68g | fiber: 17g

Fiery Couscous Salad

Prep time: 5 minutes | Cook time: 5 minutes | Serves 3

1 cup cooked or canned chickpea
½ cup dry couscous
3 tangerines
1 (2-inch) piece ginger, minced
¼ cup tahini
½ cup water
Optional Toppings:
Cinnamon
Fresh mint
Raisins

1. When using dry chickpeas, soak and cook ⅓ cup of dry chickpeas if necessary. Cook the couscous for about 5 minutes. 2. Meanwhile, add the tahini, minced ginger and water to a small airtight container or bowl. Whisk the tahini and ginger in the bowl into a smooth dressing, adding more water if necessary. Alternatively, shake the container with tahini, ginger and water until everything is thoroughly mixed, adding more water if you want a thinner and less creamy dressing. 3. Add the couscous, dressing and chickpeas to a large bowl and mix thoroughly. 4. Peel and section the tangerines and set them aside to garnish the salad. 5. Divide the salad between two bowls, garnish with the tangerines and the optional toppings, serve and enjoy! 6. Store the salad in an airtight container in the fridge, and consume within 2 days. Alternatively, store in the freezer for a maximum of 30 days and thaw at room temperature. The salad can be served cold.

Per Serving:
calories: 349 | fat: 14g | protein: 14g | carbs: 41g | fiber: 8g

Roasted Vegetable and Lentil Salad

Prep time: 15 minutes | Cook time: 25 minutes | Serves 2

4 carrots, scrubbed and trimmed
1 beet, scrubbed and trimmed
2 cups shiitake mushrooms, rinsed and dried
2 tablespoons extra-virgin olive oil (optional)
2 cloves garlic, minced
1 teaspoon garam masala
Sea salt and freshly ground black pepper, to taste (optional)
½ cup dried green lentils, soaked in water for 2 hours, or 1 cup cooked
2 cups arugula

1. To start, preheat your oven to 400ºF (205ºC) and line a baking sheet with parchment paper for easy cleanup. 2. Prepare the vegetables by halving the carrots lengthwise if they are small, or cutting them into ½-inch slices for larger ones. Quarter the beet as well. 3. In a large bowl, combine the carrots, beet, and mushrooms. Drizzle with olive oil if using, add the garlic, and sprinkle with garam masala. Toss the veggies until they are evenly coated with the spices and oil. Transfer them to the prepared baking sheet, spreading them out in a single layer. Season with salt and pepper to taste. Roast the vegetables for 20 to 25 minutes, flipping them halfway through to ensure even cooking. 4. While the vegetables roast, prepare the lentils. If using dried lentils, rinse them thoroughly and cook in a pot with 1½ cups of water. Bring to a boil, then reduce the heat and simmer until tender, approximately 15 to 20 minutes. Drain and rinse under cold water, allowing them to drain completely. If you're using canned lentils, there's no need to cook them, but be sure to rinse and drain them well. 5. When ready to serve, arrange a bed of arugula on a large platter or divide it between two plates or shallow bowls. Top the arugula with the cooked lentils and roasted vegetables. The dish can be served warm or at room temperature, making it a delightful and flavorful meal. Enjoy!

Per Serving:
calories: 381 | fat: 15g | protein: 16g | carbs: 40g | fiber: 10g

Tofu and Zoodles Dinner Salad

Prep time: 10 minutes | Cook time: 20 minutes | Serves 2

Tofu:
Olive oil cooking spray
1 (16-ounce / 454-g) package firm or extra-firm tofu
Pinch of salt (optional)
Peanut Sauce:
3 tablespoons natural peanut butter
2 tablespoons low-sodium soy sauce or gluten-free tamari
2 teaspoons maple syrup (optional)
Juice of 2 limes
Pinch red pepper flakes (optional)
Zoodles Salad:
2 small Persian cucumbers, thinly sliced
1 large carrot, peeled and julienned
5 fresh mint leaves, julienned
1 handful fresh cilantro, chopped
6 to 8 ounces (170 to 227 g) store-bought zucchini noodles (about 2 small zucchini)
2 cups mixed salad greens
1 cup shredded red cabbage

1. Prepare the Tofu: Preheat the oven to 425ºF (220ºC). Spray a sheet pan with olive oil cooking spray. 2. Drain the tofu and place it on a plate lined with a clean kitchen towel. Place another plate on top of the tofu to press out a bit more of the liquid. Pat the tofu dry with a clean kitchen towel. Cut the tofu into small cubes. 3. Spread out the tofu in a single layer on the sheet pan, sprinkle with salt (if using), and bake for 10 minutes. Using a spatula, flip the tofu and continue to bake for another 10 minutes. 4. Make the Peanut Sauce: In a medium bowl, whisk together the peanut butter, soy sauce, maple syrup, lime juice, and red pepper flakes (if using). Add water, 1 tablespoon at a time, and whisk until the sauce is thick but still pourable. Set aside. 5. Make the Salad: Put the cucumbers, carrot, mint, and cilantro in a large bowl. Add the zucchini noodles, greens, and cabbage and toss until combined. 6. To serve, portion the salad into bowls. Divide the tofu equally among the bowls and top with the peanut sauce.

Per Serving:
calories: 465 | fat: 26g | protein: 35g | carbs: 34g | fiber: 7g

Bowl

Prep time: 15 minutes | Cook time: 35 minutes | Serves 2

Roasted Vegetables:
1 sweet potato, peeled and chopped into bite-size pieces
1 parsnip, peeled and sliced into ¼-inch rounds
2 carrots, peeled and sliced into ½-inch rounds
2 tablespoons extra virgin olive oil (optional)
½ teaspoon salt (optional)
Tahini Dressing:
¼ cup tahini
1 tablespoon maple syrup
(optional)
1 tablespoon lemon juice
1 clove garlic
¼ teaspoon salt (optional)
Pinch of ground black pepper
3 tablespoons water
Assemble:
¼ cup diced red onion
½ cup chopped red cabbage
9 ounces (255 g) baby spinach
¼ cup raw shelled hempseed
1 tablespoon black or white chia seeds

Make Roasted Vegetables: 1. Preheat the oven to 375°F (190°C). 2. Place the sweet potatoes, parsnips, and carrots on a baking sheet, keeping them separated. Drizzle the oil (if desired) over the top and lightly toss, still keeping the vegetables separated. Sprinkle with salt, if desired. Bake for 30 to 35 minutes or until they can be pierced with a fork. Set aside. Make Tahini Dressing: 3. Add all the dressing ingredients to a blender and blend until smooth. Assemble: 4. Prepare the salad bowls by placing half the spinach in the bottom of each bowl. Arrange all the remaining vegetables and hempseed in a circle around the edge of the bowl. Pour half of the dressing in the center of the vegetable round. Sprinkle with the chia seeds.

Per Serving:
calories: 395 | fat: 22g | protein: 24g | carbs: 26g | fiber: 8g

Caramelized Onion Potato Salad

Prep time: 15 minutes | Cook time: 45 minutes | Serves 6

Dressing:
3 tablespoons virgin olive oil (optional)
1 tablespoon grainy mustard
1 teaspoon prepared horseradish
1 teaspoon raw agave nectar or pure maple syrup (optional)
1 tablespoon white wine vinegar
Salt and pepper, to taste (optional)
Salad:
2 teaspoons virgin olive oil
(optional)
1 large onion, cut into ¼-inch slices
1½ pounds (680 g) mini new potatoes
¼ cup chopped fresh dill
¼ cup lightly packed chopped fresh flat-leaf parsley
2 green onions, finely sliced
⅓ cup chopped dill pickles or bread-and-butter pickles
Salt and pepper, to taste (optional)

1. Make the Dressing: In a jar with a tight-fitting lid, combine the olive oil, grainy mustard, horseradish, agave nectar, white wine vinegar, salt, and pepper, if using. Tightly secure the lid, and shake the jar vigorously to combine and set aside. 2. Make the Salad: Heat the olive oil in a large pot over medium-low heat. Add the onions. Cook the onions, stirring every few minutes, for about 40 minutes or until onions are very soft and deep golden brown. There shouldn't be any dry or crispy bits of onion, and they should appear almost jammy in texture. 3. If the pan is a little dry or the onions are crisping instead of browning, lower the heat slightly and add a splash of water. After the onions are fully caramelized, scrape them into a bowl and allow them to cool. 4. While the onions are caramelizing, place the potatoes in a large saucepan over medium-high heat, and cover them with cold water by 1 inch. Bring to a boil, uncovered, and then lower the heat to a simmer. Cook the potatoes for 15 minutes or until just tender when pricked with a paring knife. 5. Drain the potatoes and run them under cold water to speed up the cooling process. Once you can handle them, cut the potatoes into quarters, wedges, or bite-sized pieces. Place the cut potatoes in a large bowl. 6. To the potatoes, add the cooled caramelized onions, along with the chopped dill, parsley, green onions, and chopped pickles. Season the salad with salt and pepper, if using. Pour the dressing over the potato salad, and toss to combine. Serve the salad cold or at room temperature.

Per Serving:
calories: 180 | fat: 9g | protein: 3g | carbs: 24g | fiber: 3g

Lentil Salad with Lemon and Fresh Herbs

Prep time: 10 minutes | Cook time: 45 minutes | Serves 4

1½ cups green lentils, rinsed
3 cups vegetable stock, or low-sodium vegetable broth
Zest of 1 lemon and juice of 2 lemons
2 cloves garlic, peeled and minced
½ cup finely chopped cilantro
2 tablespoons finely chopped mint
4 green onions (white and green parts), finely chopped, plus more for garnish
Salt and freshly ground black pepper, to taste
4 cups arugula

1. Start by placing the lentils in a medium saucepan along with the vegetable stock. Bring the mixture to a boil over high heat. Once boiling, reduce the heat to medium, cover the saucepan, and let the lentils cook for approximately 35 to 45 minutes. The lentils should become tender but not mushy. 2. After the lentils are cooked, drain them and transfer them to a large bowl. Now, add the lemon zest and juice, garlic, cilantro, mint, green onions, and season with salt and pepper. Give everything a thorough mix to combine all the flavors. 3. To serve, divide the arugula among four individual plates, creating a bed of greens. Spoon the flavorful lentil salad on top of the greens, letting the vibrant colors and textures come together beautifully. For a final touch, garnish the dish with freshly chopped green onions.

Per Serving:
calories: 277 | fat: 0g | protein: 18g | carbs: 51g | fiber: 8g

Roasted Root Vegetable Salad Bulgur Lettuce Cups

Prep time: 10 minutes | Cook time: 20 minutes | Serves 2 to 4

Sauce:
½ cup unsweetened natural peanut butter
¼ cup soy sauce
3 tablespoons seasoned rice vinegar
2 tablespoons lime juice
1 teaspoon liquid aminos
1 teaspoon sriracha
Cups:
1 cup bulgur
½ cup soy sauce
¼ cup seasoned rice vinegar
½ teaspoon garlic powder
½ teaspoon ground ginger
¼ teaspoon red pepper flakes
1 cup shredded carrots
1 cup shredded cabbage
½ cup sliced scallions, green and white parts
1 head red leaf lettuce or Bibb lettuce

Make the Sauce: 1. In a small bowl, combine the peanut butter, soy sauce, vinegar, lime juice, liquid aminos, and sriracha. Whisk until well combined. Make the Cups: 2. In a medium saucepan, cook the bulgur for about 12 minutes. Remove from the heat. Drain any excess water after cooking. 3. In a small bowl, combine the soy sauce, vinegar, garlic powder, ginger, and red pepper flakes. Mix well. 4. Add the carrots, cabbage, scallions, and soy sauce mixture to the cooked bulgur. Mix thoroughly. 5. Serve the filling scooped into individual lettuce leaves, topped with a drizzle of peanut sauce.

Per Serving:
calories: 532 | fat: 17g | protein: 25g | carbs: 79g | fiber: 18g

Chapter 9
Stews and Soups

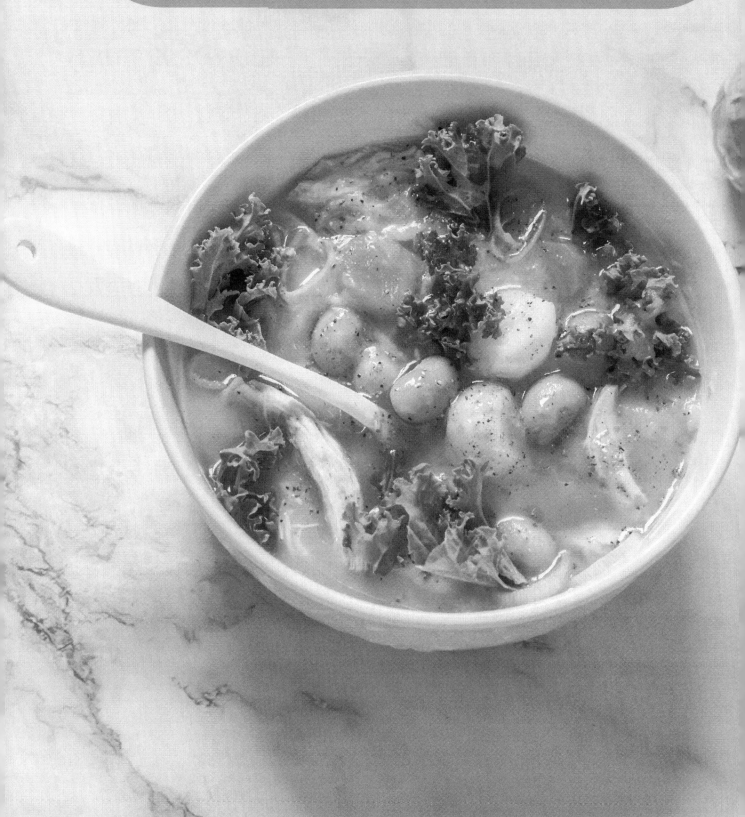

Tuscan Bean Stew

Prep time: 25 minutes | **Cook time:** 40 minutes | **Serves 6**

3 large leeks (white and light green parts), diced and rinsed
2 celery stalks, diced
2 medium carrots, peeled and diced
2 cups chopped green cabbage
1 large russet potato, peeled and diced
6 cloves garlic, peeled and minced
3 cups cooked cannellini beans
6 cups vegetable stock, or low-sodium vegetable broth
½ cup chopped basil
Salt and freshly ground black pepper, to taste

1. In a large saucepan, combine the leeks, celery, and carrots, and sauté over medium heat for about 10 minutes. If needed, add water 1 to 2 tablespoons at a time to prevent the vegetables from sticking to the pan. 2. To the sautéed vegetables, add the cabbage, potato, garlic, beans, and vegetable stock. Bring the soup to a boil over high heat, then lower the heat to medium and cook, uncovered, for approximately 30 minutes until the potatoes become tender. Stir in the basil and season the soup with salt and pepper to taste.

Per Serving:
calories: 128 | fat: 0g | protein: 3g | carbs: 29g | fiber: 4g

Minestrone

Prep time: 30 minutes | **Cook time:** 55 minutes | **Serves 8 to 10**

1 large onion, peeled and chopped
2 large carrots, peeled and chopped
2 celery stalks, chopped
4 cloves garlic, peeled and minced
8 cups vegetable stock, or low-sodium vegetable broth
2 tablespoons nutritional yeast (optional)
1 (28-ounce / 794-g) can diced tomatoes
2 teaspoons oregano
2 medium red-skin potatoes, scrubbed and cubed
4 cups packed chopped kale, ribs removed before chopping
½ cup uncooked brown basmati rice
6 cups cooked cannellini beans, or 3 (15-ounce / 425-g) cans, drained and rinsed
Salt and freshly ground black pepper, to taste
1 cup finely chopped basil

1. In a large saucepan over medium heat, sauté the onion, carrots, and celery for 10 minutes. To prevent sticking, add water 1 to 2 tablespoons at a time as needed.
2. Stir in the garlic and cook for an additional minute. Add the vegetable stock, and if using, nutritional yeast, tomatoes, oregano, potatoes, kale, and rice. Bring the mixture to a boil over high heat, then reduce the heat to medium-low and let it simmer for 30 minutes. 3. After 30 minutes, add the beans and continue to simmer for an additional 15 minutes or until the rice is tender. Season the soup with salt and pepper to taste, and then stir in the fresh basil.

Per Serving:
calories: 118 | fat: 2g | protein: 5g | carbs: 24g | fiber: 7g

Ful Nabed (Egyptian Fava Bean Soup)

Prep time: 25 minutes | **Cook time:** 40 minutes | **Serves 4 to 6**

1 large yellow onion, peeled and diced
1 medium carrot, peeled and diced
1 celery stalk, thinly sliced
4 cloves garlic, peeled
2 teaspoons cumin seeds, toasted and ground
1 tablespoon sweet paprika
2 bay leaves
1 large tomato, finely chopped
6 cups vegetable stock, or low-sodium vegetable broth
3 cups cooked fava beans
¼ teaspoon cayenne pepper, or to taste
¼ cup finely chopped parsley
Zest and juice of 1 lemon
2 tablespoons finely chopped mint
Salt, to taste (optional)

1. In a large pot, sauté the onion, carrot, and celery over medium heat for 10 minutes. To prevent sticking, add water 1 to 2 tablespoons at a time as needed. Stir in the garlic, cumin, paprika, bay leaves, and tomato, and cook for an additional 5 minutes. Pour in the vegetable stock and add the fava beans. Cover the pot and let it simmer for 20 minutes. 2. Stir in the cayenne pepper, parsley, lemon zest and juice, and mint. Cook for another 5 minutes, allowing the flavors to meld together. Season with salt to taste, if desired.

Per Serving:
calories: 99 | fat: 0g | protein: 6g | carbs: 21g | fiber: 6g

Carrot Ginger Soup

Prep time: 15 minutes | **Cook time:** 25 minutes | **Serves 6**

3 tablespoons water
1 cup diced red, white, or yellow onion
1 teaspoon minced garlic
2 tablespoons minced ginger
3 cups chopped carrots
2 cups chopped russet potatoes
4 cups vegetable broth
Salt and pepper, to taste (optional)

1. Begin by heating water in a large pot over medium-high heat. 2. Once the water is hot, add the onion, garlic, and ginger to the pot. Sauté the ingredients for about 2 to 3 minutes, or until the onion turns translucent and tender. 3. Next, include the carrots, potatoes, and broth in the pot. Allow the mixture to cook for approximately 20 minutes or until the carrots and potatoes become tender. 4. Remove the pot from the heat. Now, using an immersion blender, carefully purée the soup until it reaches a smooth and creamy consistency. Alternatively, you can use a regular blender, working in batches. 5. Finally, season the soup with salt and pepper to taste, ensuring it has just the right balance of flavors.

Per Serving:
calories: 80 | fat: 0g | protein: 2g | carbs: 18g | fiber: 3g

Coconut Watercress Soup

Prep time: 10 minutes | **Cook time:** 15 minutes | Makes 4 bowls

- 1 teaspoon coconut oil (optional)
- 1 onion, diced
- 2 cups fresh or frozen peas
- 4 cups water or vegetable stock
- 1 cup fresh watercress, chopped
- 1 tablespoon fresh mint, chopped
- Pinch sea salt (optional)
- Pinch freshly ground black pepper
- ¾ cup coconut milk

1. If using coconut oil, melt it in a large pot over medium-high heat. Add the onion and sauté until softened, which takes about 5 minutes. Then, add the peas and water to the pot. 2. Bring the mixture to a boil, and then reduce the heat. Add the watercress, mint, and season with salt and pepper (if desired). Cover the pot and let it simmer for 5 minutes. 3. After the simmering, stir in the coconut milk. To achieve a smooth consistency, transfer the soup to a blender or use an immersion blender to purée it until it becomes creamy and velvety.

Per Serving: (1 bowl)
calories: 155 | fat: 12g | protein: 3g | carbs: 10g | fiber: 3g

Miso Noodle Soup with Shiitake Mushrooms

Prep time: 5 minutes | **Cook time:** 25 minutes | Serves 4 to 6

- 1 (8-ounce / 227-g) package brown rice noodles
- 4 cups vegetable broth
- 2 cups water
- 1 (5-ounce / 142-g) package shiitake mushrooms, cut into ¼-inch-thick slices
- 3 scallions, green and white parts, thinly sliced on a bias (about ½ cup)
- 3 garlic cloves, sliced
- 3 or 4 (¼-inch) slices unpeeled fresh ginger
- 8 ounces (227 g) bok choy
- 2 tablespoons red miso paste
- 1 tablespoon soy sauce

1. Begin by cooking the noodles for approximately 5 minutes until they are tender and ready. 2. In a generously sized Dutch oven or saucepan, combine the broth, water, mushrooms, scallions, garlic, and ginger. Cover the pot and bring the mixture to a boil over high heat. 3. Once boiling, reduce the heat to low, cover the pot again, and let it simmer for 15 minutes, allowing the flavors to meld. 4. Carefully uncover the pot, increase the heat to medium, and add the bok choy. Continue to simmer for 3 minutes, or until the bok choy reaches a delightful crisp-tender texture. . Next, add the cooked noodles to the broth and vegetables, gently heating everything through.
6. Remove the pot from the heat, and now it's time to add the miso and soy sauce. Stir diligently until the miso completely dissolves, enriching the soup with its savory essence. 7. Finally, remove the ginger from the soup, as its essence has infused the broth. Your delicious and comforting noodle soup with mushrooms and bok choy is now ready to be savored and enjoyed!

Per Serving:
calories: 396 | fat: 3g | protein: 13g | carbs: 80g | fiber: 8g

Sick Day Soup

Prep time: 15 minutes | **Cook time:** 25 minutes | Serves 6

- 3 tablespoons water
- ½ cup diced red, white, or yellow onion
- 2 carrots, thinly sliced
- 2 ribs celery, thinly sliced
- ⅓ cup grated or finely chopped ginger
- 8 cloves garlic, peeled and halved
- 5 cups vegetable broth
- 4 to 5 tablespoons lemon juice
- 1 (14-ounce / 397-g) block extra-firm tofu, pressed and cut into ½-inch cubes
- ⅓ cup hot sauce
- 1 (8-ounce / 227-g) package rice noodles

1. Heat water in a large pot over medium-high heat. 2. Add onion, carrots, celery, ginger, and garlic to the pot. Sauté for about 10 minutes, until the onion turns tender and translucent. 3. Pour in the broth and add lemon juice, tofu, and hot sauce.
4. Introduce the noodles and cook according to the instructions provided on the package.

Per Serving:
calories: 131 | fat: 5g | protein: 9g | carbs: 16g | fiber: 1g

Potato, Carrot, and Mushroom Stew

Prep time: 5 minutes | **Cook time:** 25 minutes | Serves 4 to 6

- 4 cups vegetable broth
- 1½ pounds (680 g) yellow potatoes, cut into ½-inch dice (about 4 cups)
- 1 cup frozen carrots
- 1 cup frozen pearl onions
- 2 tablespoons tomato paste
- 3 strips dried porcini mushrooms, chopped (about 2 tablespoons)
- 1 tablespoon onion powder
- ½ teaspoon dried thyme
- ¼ teaspoon garlic powder
- 1 bay leaf
- ½ cup frozen peas
- 2 tablespoons red miso paste
- 1 tablespoon balsamic vinegar

1. In a spacious Dutch oven or saucepan, bring together the broth, potatoes, carrots, onions, tomato paste, mushrooms, onion powder, thyme, garlic powder, and bay leaf. Let the mixture reach a boil over high heat. 2. Once boiling, lower the heat to a gentle simmer. Cover the pot and let it cook for approximately 15 minutes, or until the potatoes become tender and easily yield to a knife. Remove the pot from the heat. 3. Stir in the peas, miso, and vinegar until the miso has fully dissolved, infusing the soup with wonderful flavors. 4. Before serving, be sure to remove the bay leaf, and then enjoy the delightful and comforting soup immediately.

Per Serving:
calories: 183 | fat: 1g | protein: 8g | carbs: 36g | fiber: 5g

Potato, Corn and Bean Soup

Prep time: 30 minutes | Cook time: 35 minutes | Serves 8

1 large yellow onion, peeled and diced
3 cloves garlic, peeled and minced
1 tablespoon minced thyme
8 cups vegetable stock, or low-sodium vegetable broth
1 pound (454 g) red-skin potatoes (7 to 9 small), scrubbed and cut into ½-inch cubes
1 pound (454 g) green beans, trimmed and cut into ½-inch pieces
6 ears corn, kernels removed (about 3½ cups)
4 cups cooked navy beans, or 2 (15-ounce / 425-g) cans, drained and rinsed
Salt and freshly ground black pepper, to taste

1. Take a large pot and place the onion in it. Begin sautéing the onion over medium heat for about 10 minutes. To prevent sticking, add 1 to 2 tablespoons of water as needed. 2. After the onion turns soft and translucent, add the garlic and thyme, and cook for an additional minute. Next, introduce the vegetable stock, potatoes, green beans, and corn to the pot. Cover it and let the ingredients cook over medium heat for 15 minutes. 3. Finally, add the navy beans, and season the stew with salt and pepper to taste. Continue cooking for another 10 minutes until the vegetables reach the desired tenderness. Now, your flavorful and nourishing vegetable stew is ready to be enjoyed!

Per Serving:
calories: 258 | fat: 1g | protein: 12g | carbs: 53g | fiber: 15g

"Don't Waste the Good Stuff" Squash Soup

Prep time: 15 minutes | Cook time: 30 minutes | Serves 6

2 (2-pound / 907-g) butternut squash
Salt and black pepper (optional)
1 large yellow onion, peeled and quartered
2 carrots, roughly chopped
1 celery rib, roughly chopped
3 garlic cloves, chopped
2 bay leaves
2 tablespoons fresh sage, chopped
3 sprigs fresh thyme, leaves stripped and stems discarded
2 sprigs fresh rosemary, leaves stripped and chopped fine, stems discarded
6 cups water
2 cups cooked white beans
2 tablespoons gluten-free mild white miso

1. Set your oven to a temperature of 425ºF (220ºC) and line a baking sheet with parchment paper for easy cleanup. 2. Begin by slicing the squash in half and removing the seeds and innards. Transfer these parts to a large stockpot. Sprinkle the squash halves with salt (if desired) and pepper, then place them cut side down on the prepared baking sheet. 3. Bake the squash in the oven until it becomes fork-tender, which should take about 25 minutes. Once done, take the baking sheet out of the oven and carefully flip the squash halves, so the cut side faces upward to cool more quickly. 4. While the squash is baking, it's time to prepare the stockpot. Add the onion, carrots, celery, garlic, bay leaves, sage, thyme, rosemary, and water to the stockpot along with the squash innards and seeds. Bring everything to a boil, then lower the heat to medium-low. Let it cook uncovered until the squash finishes baking. Afterward, remove the stockpot from the heat and discard the bay leaves.
5. Once the squash is cool enough to handle, scoop out the flesh and transfer it to a blender. Add the contents of the stockpot and the white beans (you might need to do this in batches to fit everything). Blend the mixture until smooth, creating a luscious, creamy soup. Pour the blended soup back into the stockpot. 6. Whisk in the miso, then season the soup with salt and pepper to your taste preferences. Now it's ready to be served and enjoyed, a delightful and nourishing treat!

Per Serving:
calories: 243 | fat: 1g | protein: 10g | carbs: 54g | fiber: 11g

Weeknight Root Vegetable Dhal

Prep time: 20 minutes | Cook time: 50 minutes | Serves 4

1 cup red split lentils, rinsed
1 cup finely diced root vegetables of your choice
1 small yellow onion, finely diced
1 cup cherry or grape tomatoes, halved
4 cloves garlic, minced
1 (2-inch) piece of fresh ginger, peeled and minced
1 teaspoon ground turmeric
Pinch of dried chili flakes
3½ cups filtered water
Salt and pepper, to taste (optional)
2 tablespoons virgin coconut oil (optional)
½ teaspoon cumin seeds
½ teaspoon coriander seeds
½ teaspoon mustard seeds
⅓ cup chopped fresh cilantro leaves, for garnish
Lemon wedges, for serving

1. To a medium soup pot, add the rinsed lentils, diced root vegetables, diced onion, tomatoes, garlic, ginger, turmeric, and chili flakes. Pour the water into the pot and give everything a little stir. 2. Place the pot on the stove over medium heat. Bring to a boil and then simmer for about 40 minutes, whisking the dal often. Toward the end, the lentils should be completely broken down. In the last 10 minutes of cooking, whisk the dal vigorously to encourage the breaking down of the lentils. It should appear quite soupy. Season the dal generously with salt and pepper, if using. Keep warm. 3. Heat the coconut oil in a small sauté pan over medium-high heat. Add the cumin seeds, coriander seeds, and mustard seeds. Once the seeds are fragrant and popping, remove from the heat. 4. Gently spoon the toasted spice oil (with the whole spices) on top of the dal. You can lightly stir it in if you like. You can also portion the dal out first and then spoon the spice oil on top if you like. Garnish the dal with the chopped cilantro. Serve the dal hot with lemon wedges.

Per Serving: (1 cup)
calories: 270 | fat: 8g | protein: 13g | carbs: 40g | fiber: 8g

Lentil Soup

Prep time: 5 minutes | Cook time: 25 minutes | Serves 2 to 4

4 cups vegetable broth	½ teaspoon ground cumin
1 cup dried green or brown lentils, rinsed	½ teaspoon smoked paprika
	¼ teaspoon garlic powder
2 teaspoon onion powder	¼ teaspoon ground coriander
1 teaspoon dried parsley	1 bay leaf

1. In a Dutch oven or saucepan, gather the broth, lentils, onion powder, parsley, cumin, paprika, garlic powder, coriander, and bay leaf. Let them come together as they start to boil over high heat. 2. Lower the heat to a gentle medium-low setting, cover the pot, and let the flavors simmer and meld for about 20 minutes until the lentils become tender and delightful. Once they're cooked to perfection, remove the pot from the heat. 3. It's time to take out the bay leaf, as it has worked its magic in infusing the dish with wonderful aromas and flavors. Serve the lentil goodness immediately and savor each spoonful of this heartwarming meal!

Per Serving:
calories: 100 | fat: 3g | protein: 11g | carbs: 7g | fiber: 1g

Roasted Red Pepper and Butternut Squash Soup

Prep time: 10 minutes | Cook time: 40 to 50 minutes | Makes 6 bowls

1 small butternut squash	broth
1 tablespoon olive oil (optional)	Zest and juice of 1 lime
	1 to 2 tablespoons tahini
1 teaspoon sea salt (optional)	Pinch cayenne pepper
2 red bell peppers	½ teaspoon ground coriander
1 yellow onion	½ teaspoon ground cumin
1 head garlic	Toasted squash seeds (optional)
2 cups water or vegetable	

1. Preheat your oven to 350°F (180°C). 2. To prepare the squash for roasting, cut it in half lengthwise, remove the seeds, and pierce the flesh with a fork. If desired, you can reserve the seeds. Rub a small amount of oil over the flesh and skin, then sprinkle with a bit of sea salt. Place the halves skin-side down in a large baking dish and place it in the preheated oven while you work on the other vegetables.
3. Treat the peppers the same way, cutting them in half, removing the seeds, and rubbing with oil. For the onion, slice it in half and rub oil on the exposed faces. For the garlic, slice off the top, exposing the cloves, and rub oil on the exposed flesh.
4. After the squash has roasted for 20 minutes, add the peppers, onion, and garlic to the baking dish, and continue roasting for another 20 minutes. If you like, you can also toast the reserved squash seeds by placing them in a separate baking dish about 10 to 15 minutes before the vegetables are finished. Keep a close eye on the seeds to avoid burning them. 5. Once the vegetables are cooked, remove them from the oven and allow them to cool before handling. The squash should be very soft when poked with a fork. 6. Scoop the flesh out of the squash skin and place it in a large pot if you have an immersion blender, or in a regular blender. Roughly chop the roasted peppers, remove the onion skin and chop it roughly, and squeeze the garlic cloves out of the head, all adding them to the pot or blender. Add water, lime zest, lime juice, and tahini. Puree the soup until smooth, adjusting the consistency with more water if needed. 7. Season the soup with salt (if using), cayenne, coriander, and cumin. Serve the soup garnished with toasted squash seeds if desired. Enjoy!

Per Serving: (1 bowl)
calories: 58 | fat: 3g | protein: 1g | carbs: 5g | fiber: 0g

Golden Split Pea Soup

Prep time: 10 minutes | Cook time: 3 to 4 hours | Serves 5 to 7

1 medium onion, diced	4 cups low-sodium vegetable broth or water
3 carrots, diced	
3 celery stalks, diced	1 bay leaf
3 garlic cloves, crushed	¾ teaspoon ground cumin
1 cup yellow split peas, rinsed and stones removed	¾ teaspoon ground turmeric
	½ teaspoon dry mustard
1 yellow potato (about ⅓ pound / 136 g), unpeeled and cubed	Ground black pepper
	Salt (optional)

1. In the slow cooker, combine the onion, carrots, celery, garlic, peas, potato, broth, bay leaf, cumin, turmeric, mustard, pepper, and salt (if desired). Cover and cook on High for 3 to 4 hours or on Low for 7 to 8 hours. 2. Once cooked, remove and discard the bay leaf. Use an immersion blender or countertop blender to fully purée the soup before serving.

Per Serving:
calories: 207 | fat: 1g | protein: 11g | carbs: 40g | fiber: 13g

Italian Lentil Soup

Prep time: 10 minutes | Cook time: 3 to 4 hours | Serves 6 to 8

1 medium onion, diced	1 (28-ounce / 794-g) can no-salt-added crushed tomatoes
3 garlic cloves, minced	
2 carrots, diced	8 cups store-bought low-sodium vegetable broth
2 celery stalks, diced	
1 pound (454 g, about 2⅓ cups) dried green or brown lentils, rinsed and sorted	1 tablespoon Italian seasoning
	Ground black pepper
	Salt (optional)

1. Put the onion, garlic, carrots, celery, lentils, tomatoes, broth, Italian seasoning, pepper, and salt (if using) in the slow cooker. 2. Cover and cook on High for 3 to 4 hours or on Low for 7 to 8 hours.

Per Serving:
calories: 354 | fat: 1g | protein: 20g | carbs: 67g | fiber: 34g

White Bean, Butternut Squash, and Kale Soup

Prep time: 15 minutes | Cook time: 15 minutes | Serves 4

½ medium butternut squash, peeled, seeded, and cut into small pieces (about 2 cups)
4 cups water, divided
1 bunch kale, stemmed, leaves chopped small
2 (15-ounce / 425-g) cans cannellini beans, drained and rinsed
1½ teaspoons salt (optional)
1½ teaspoons onion powder
1 teaspoon garlic powder
½ teaspoon smoked paprika
1 teaspoon red miso paste
Red pepper flakes

1. In a medium saucepan, combine the squash with 2 cups of water and bring it to a boil over high heat. Reduce the heat to medium and cook until the squash is fork-tender, approximately 5 minutes. 2. Using a slotted spoon, transfer half of the softened squash to a blender, along with the remaining 2 cups of water, and blend until smooth. Return the blended mixture to the pot. 3. Add the kale, cannellini beans, salt (if desired), onion powder, garlic powder, and smoked paprika to the pot and bring it to a boil. Cook until the kale is tender, about 5 minutes. 4. Remove the pot from the heat, add the miso, and stir well until the miso dissolves. Spoon the soup into bowls and sprinkle with red pepper flakes.

Per Serving:
calories: 273 | fat: 2g | protein: 16g | carbs: 53g | fiber: 19g

Caribbean Coconut Collards and Sweet Potatoes

Prep time: 20 minutes | Cook time: 35 minutes | Serves 4

1 tablespoon coconut oil (optional)
1 yellow onion, diced
3 garlic cloves, chopped
½ teaspoon crushed red pepper
2 bunches collard greens, stemmed, leaves chopped into 1-inch squares
1 large sweet potato, peeled and diced
1 (15-ounce / 425-g) can red kidney beans or chickpeas, drained and rinsed
1 (14½-ounce / 411-g) can diced tomatoes with juice
1½ cups water
½ cup light or full-fat coconut milk
Salt and black pepper (optional)

1. In a large, deep skillet, melt the oil (if using) over medium heat. Add the onion, garlic, and crushed red pepper, and cook for 3 minutes. Stir in the collards and sweet potato, then add the beans, tomatoes with their juice, water, and coconut milk. 2. Bring the mixture to a gentle boil, then reduce the heat to medium-low. Cover the skillet and cook until the collards and sweet potato are tender, approximately 30 minutes. 3. Season the dish with salt and pepper to taste. Serve, if desired.

Per Serving:
calories: 300 | fat: 12g | protein: 12g | carbs: 40g | fiber: 11g

Quick and Easy Thai Vegetable Stew

Prep time: 20 minutes | Cook time: 20 minutes | Serves 4

1 medium yellow onion, peeled and diced small
2 cloves garlic, peeled and minced
2 teaspoons grated ginger
2 teaspoons Thai red chili paste, or to taste
Zest and juice of 1 lime
1 serrano chile, minced (for less heat, remove the seeds)
2 tablespoons low-sodium soy sauce, or to taste
1 (14-ounce / 397-g) can lite coconut milk
1 cup vegetable stock, or low-sodium vegetable broth
3 cups mixed vegetables of your choice, such as edamame, water chestnuts, carrots, broccoli florets, or sugar snap peas
½ cup chopped cilantro
2 tablespoons minced mint

1. In a large saucepan, place the onion and sauté over medium-high heat for 7 to 8 minutes until it becomes tender and starts to brown. To prevent sticking, add water 1 to 2 tablespoons at a time. 2. Stir in the garlic, ginger, chili paste, lime zest and juice, and serrano chile, and cook for 30 seconds. Next, add the soy sauce, coconut milk, vegetable stock, and mixed vegetables. Reduce the heat to medium and cook for 10 minutes until the vegetables are tender. Finally, stir in the cilantro and mint before serving.

Per Serving:
calories: 336 | fat: 27g | protein: 5g | carbs: 21g | fiber: 7g

Curried Zucchini Soup

Prep time: 10 minutes | Cook time: 3 to 4 hours | Serves 4 to 6

1 medium onion, chopped
3 garlic cloves, minced
3 medium zucchini (about 1½ pounds / 680 g), chopped into 1-inch pieces
2 yellow potatoes (about ⅔ pound / 272 g), unpeeled and chopped
5 cups store-bought low-sodium vegetable broth
1 tablespoon curry powder
Ground black pepper
Salt (optional)

1. Combine the onion, garlic, zucchini, potatoes, broth, curry powder, pepper, and salt (if desired) in the slow cooker. Cover and cook on High for 3 to 4 hours or on Low for 6 to 7 hours. 2. Prior to serving, use an immersion blender to blend the soup until smooth directly in the slow cooker. Alternatively, transfer the contents in batches to a regular blender, blending carefully starting on low and gradually increasing the speed to avoid any hot soup splatters.

Per Serving:
calories: 119 | fat: 1g | protein: 5g | carbs: 25g | fiber: 5g

Chipotle Black Bean Soup

Prep time: 30 minutes | **Cook time:** 35 minutes | **Serves 4**

- 1 large yellow onion, peeled and diced
- 1 large green bell pepper, seeded and diced
- 3 cloves garlic, peeled and minced
- 1 tablespoon cumin seeds, toasted and ground
- 1 teaspoon dried Mexican oregano, toasted
- 1 teaspoon coriander seeds, toasted and ground
- 1 dried chipotle pepper, halved, toasted in a dry skillet for 2 to 3 minutes, soaked in cool water for 15 minutes, and chopped
- 1 cup orange juice
- Zest of 1 orange
- 4 cups cooked black beans, or 2 (15-ounce / 425-g) cans, drained and rinsed
- Salt and freshly ground black pepper, to taste

1. In a large pan, place the onion and green pepper and sauté over medium heat for 7 to 8 minutes. To prevent sticking, add water 1 to 2 tablespoons at a time. 2. Stir in the garlic, cumin, oregano, coriander, and chipotle pepper, and cook for 2 minutes. Add the orange juice, orange zest, beans, and enough water to cover the beans by 3 inches. Bring the soup to a boil over high heat. Then, reduce the heat to medium and cook, covered, for 25 minutes. Finally, season with salt and pepper to taste.

Per Serving:
calories: 293 | fat: 1g | protein: 17g | carbs: 54g | fiber: 17g

Small-Batch Roasted Soup

Prep time: 10 minutes | **Cook time:** 40 minutes | **Serves 2**

- 2 cups chopped seasonal vegetables
- 1 small onion, chopped
- 1 clove garlic, peeled
- 2 teaspoons virgin olive oil (optional)
- Salt and pepper, to taste
- (optional)
- 1 cup cooked beans
- 1½ cups vegetable stock
- 2 teaspoons fresh lemon juice
- Serve:
- Bread or cooked rice, millet, or quinoa

1. Preheat your oven to 400ºF (205ºC). 2. On a baking sheet lined with parchment paper, toss the chopped seasonal vegetables, onions, and garlic clove with olive oil, and season with salt and pepper if desired. Make sure the vegetables are evenly coated with the oil, then place the baking sheet in the preheated oven. 3. Roast the vegetables until the onions are lightly browned, and your seasonal vegetables are becoming tender. Asparagus or broccoli may take around 15 to 20 minutes, while sweet potatoes and squash could take about 35 minutes. Remove the baking sheet from the oven once they are cooked to your desired tenderness. 4. Transfer the roasted vegetables into a blender and add the beans, vegetable stock, and lemon juice. Gradually increase the blender speed to high and blend until the mixture becomes smooth and creamy. 5. Pour the blended soup into a medium saucepan and bring it to a boil, leaving the saucepan uncovered. Taste the soup and adjust the seasoning as needed. Serve the soup hot, accompanied by bread on the side or with cooked rice, millet, or quinoa on top. Enjoy!

Per Serving:
calories: 110 | fat: 5g | protein: 4g | carbs: 15g | fiber: 5g

Fancy Instant Ramen Soup

Prep time: 10 minutes | **Cook time:** 20 minutes | **Serves 4**

- 6 cups water
- ½ cup chopped frozen broccoli
- ½ cup frozen mixed vegetables
- ½ teaspoon minced garlic
- 3 (3-ounce / 85-g) packages instant ramen noodles

1. In a large pot over high heat, bring the water to a boil. 2. Add the broccoli, mixed vegetables, and garlic. Boil for 5 minutes. 3. Stir in the ramen noodles and cook the noodles according to the directions on the package, but use only two of the three seasoning packets. 4. Remove from the heat. Serve immediately.

Per Serving:
calories: 301 | fat: 11g | protein: 8g | carbs: 42g | fiber: 4g

Lentil Soup with Cauliflower, Potatoes and Spinach

Prep time: 25 minutes | **Cook time:** 1 hour | **Serves 8 to 10**

- 1 large onion, peeled and chopped
- 6 cloves garlic, peeled and minced
- 2 bay leaves
- 2 teaspoons curry powder, or to taste
- ½ teaspoon turmeric
- Pinch ground nutmeg
- 1 (15-ounce / 425-g) can diced tomatoes
- 1 cup green lentils, rinsed
- 2 large waxy potatoes, scrubbed and cut into ½-inch dice
- 1 small head cauliflower, cut into florets
- 6 cups finely chopped spinach leaves
- 2 tablespoons minced cilantro
- Zest and juice of 1 lemon
- Salt and freshly ground black pepper, to taste

1. In a large pot, sauté the onions over medium heat for about 10 minutes. To prevent sticking, add water 1 to 2 tablespoons at a time. Add the garlic and cook for another minute. Then, stir in the bay leaves, curry powder, turmeric, and nutmeg, and cook for an additional minute. Mix in the tomatoes and cook for about 3 minutes. Next, add the lentils and 6 cups of water, and bring it to a boil over high heat. Reduce the heat to medium, cover the pot, and let it cook for 30 minutes. After that, include the potatoes and cauliflower, and continue cooking until the lentils are tender, approximately 15 more minutes. 2. Finally, add the spinach, cilantro, and lemon zest and juice to the pot. Season with salt and pepper to taste.

Per Serving:
calories: 130 | fat: 0g | protein: 7g | carbs: 25g | fiber: 5g

Spanish Chickpea Stew

Prep time: 30 minutes | Cook time: 40 minutes | Serves 4

1 medium onion, peeled and diced small
1 green bell pepper, seeded and diced small
2 cloves garlic, peeled and minced
1 teaspoon cumin seeds, toasted and ground
1 teaspoon sweet paprika
½ teaspoon smoked paprika
1 bay leaf
1 large tomato, diced small
3 medium Yukon Gold potatoes (about 1 pound / 454 g), cut into ½-inch dice
5 cups vegetable stock, or low-sodium vegetable broth
2 cups cooked chickpeas, or 1 (15-ounce / 425-g) can, drained and rinsed
1 medium bunch Swiss chard, ribs removed, chopped
Salt and freshly ground black pepper, to taste

1. Place the onion and pepper in a large pot and sauté over medium heat for 10 minutes. Add water 1 to 2 tablespoons at a time to keep the vegetables from sticking to the pot. 2. Add the garlic, cumin, both kinds of paprika, and bay leaf and cook for 1 minute. Stir in the tomato and cook for 3 minutes. Add the potatoes, vegetable stock, and chickpeas and bring the pot to a boil over high heat. 3. Reduce the heat to medium and cook, covered, for 20 minutes, or until the potatoes are tender. Add the Swiss chard, season with salt and pepper, and cook, covered, until the chard wilts, about 5 minutes.

Per Serving:
calories: 304 | fat: 2g | protein: 12g | carbs: 60g | fiber: 11g

Coconut Curry Soup

Prep time: 25 minutes | Cook time: 20 minutes | Serves 6

3 tablespoons water
¾ cup diced red, white, or yellow onion
1½ teaspoons minced garlic
1 cup diced green or red bell pepper
1 (14½-ounce / 411-g) can diced tomatoes with their juices
1 (15-ounce / 425-g) can chickpeas, drained and rinsed
4 cups vegetable broth
1½ teaspoons ground cumin
2½ teaspoons curry powder
1 (13½-ounce / 383-g) can full-fat coconut milk
½ cup cooked brown rice
Salt and pepper, to taste (optional)
Optional Toppings:
Red chili flakes
Minced cilantro

1. Place a large pot over medium heat and heat the water. 2. Add the onion, garlic, and bell pepper to the pot. Cook and stir occasionally for about 5 minutes, until the vegetables become tender. 3. Stir in the tomatoes, chickpeas, broth, cumin, and curry powder. Bring the mixture to a boil, then reduce the heat to low and let it simmer gently for 10 minutes, stirring occasionally. 4. After 10 minutes, add the coconut milk and brown rice to the pot. Continue cooking for an additional 5 minutes, stirring occasionally. 5. Season with salt and pepper to taste, if desired. Serve and enjoy your flavorful dish!

Per Serving:
calories: 126 | fat: 2g | protein: 5g | carbs: 24g | fiber: 6g

Chilean Bean Stew

Prep time: 20 minutes | Cook time: 35 minutes | Serves 4

1 large yellow onion, peeled and diced small
4 cloves garlic, peeled and minced
1 medium butternut squash (about 1 pound / 454 g), peeled, halved, seeded, and cut into ½-inch pieces
2 cups cooked pinto beans, or 1 (15-ounce / 425-g) can, drained and rinsed
6 ears corn, kernels removed (about 3½ cups)
Salt and freshly ground black pepper, to taste
1 cup finely chopped basil

1. Place the onion in a large saucepan and sauté over medium heat for 10 minutes. Add water 1 to 2 tablespoons at a time to keep the onion from sticking to the pan. 2. Add the garlic, squash, beans, corn, and 2 cups of water and cook for 25 minutes, or until the squash is tender. Season with salt and pepper and stir in the basil.

Per Serving:
calories: 305 | fat: 2g | protein: 15g | carbs: 65g | fiber: 14g

Winter Squash Soup

Prep time: 15 minutes | Cook time: 30 minutes | Makes 2½ quarts

2 tablespoons extra-virgin coconut oil (optional)
1 medium yellow onion, diced
3 large garlic cloves, finely chopped
2 teaspoons fine sea salt, plus more to taste (optional)
1 large winter squash, halved, seeded, peeled, and cut into 1-inch cubes
5 cups filtered water
Freshly ground black pepper
Tamari (optional)

1. Heat the oil in a large pot over medium-high heat. Add the onion and cook for 6 to 8 minutes until it starts to brown. Stir in the garlic and salt (if using) and cook for an additional 3 to 4 minutes until the garlic becomes fragrant and golden. Add the squash and enough water (almost to the top of the chopped squash) to cover it. Increase the heat and bring to a boil, then cover the pot, reduce the heat to low, and let it simmer for 12 to 15 minutes until the squash becomes tender. To check if it's ready, press a piece of squash against the side of the pot; it should crush easily with slight pressure. Remove from heat, add pepper to taste, and allow it to cool slightly.
2. In batches, transfer the soup to an upright blender (filling it no more than two-thirds full) and blend on high speed until smooth and velvety. Pour the blended soup into a large bowl or another pot. Season with additional salt, pepper, and tamari (if using) to taste. Serve the soup warm. You can store any leftovers in jars in the fridge for up to 5 days, or freeze them for up to 3 months.

Per Serving: (½ quart)
calories: 93 | fat: 6g | protein: 1g | carbs: 12g | fiber: 2g

Lentil Rice Soup

Prep time: 10 minutes | Cook time: 30 minutes | Serves 4

- ⅓ cup dry quick-cooking brown rice
- ⅔ cup dried green lentils
- 1 cup canned or fresh tomato cubes
- 3 cups vegetable stock
- ¼ cup tahini
- Optional Toppings:
- Fresh chili slices
- Fresh cilantro
- Green peppercorns

1. Place a large pot over medium-high heat and pour in the vegetable stock along with the green lentils. 2. Bring the stock to a boil, then reduce the heat to medium. 3. Allow the lentils to cook for approximately 15 minutes, keeping the pot uncovered. Occasionally, skim off any foam that may form and give the pot a gentle stir. 4. Next, add the brown rice and lower the heat to a simmer. Cover the pot with a lid and let it simmer for an additional 10 minutes. 5. Stir in the tomato cubes and tahini, making sure everything is well combined. Let the soup simmer for another 5 minutes. 6. Turn off the heat and allow the soup to cool down for 5 minutes. 7. Divide the soup into two bowls, serve with optional toppings, and enjoy! 8. If there are any leftovers, store the soup in an airtight container in the fridge and consume within 2 days. Alternatively, you can store it in the freezer for up to 60 days. To reheat, use either a pot or the microwave.

Per Serving:
calories: 284 | fat: 10g | protein: 15g | carbs: 33g | fiber: 12g

Lima Bean Stew

Prep time: 20 minutes | Cook time: 1 hour 15 minutes | Serves 6

- 1½ cups dried lima beans, soaked for 8 to 10 hours (or overnight) and drained
- 2 bay leaves
- 4 whole cloves
- 4 cloves garlic, peeled
- 1 large onion, peeled and chopped
- 2 celery stalks, chopped
- 2 medium carrots, peeled and chopped
- 1 green bell pepper, seeded and sliced
- 1 teaspoon thyme leaves
- ¼ cup tomato paste
- Salt and freshly ground black pepper, to taste

1. Place the soaked lima beans in a pot with 4 cups water and add the bay leaves, cloves, and garlic. Simmer for 1 hour, or until the beans are just tender, adding more water as needed to cover the beans well. Remove the bay leaves, cloves, and garlic. 2. While the beans are cooking, place the onion, celery, and carrots in a large saucepan and sauté over medium heat for 10 minutes. Add water 1 to 2 tablespoons at a time to keep the vegetables from sticking to the pan. Add the green pepper and thyme and cook for 4 minutes. Add the tomato paste and cook for 1 minute. 3. Add the vegetable mixture to the cooked beans and cook for 15 minutes over medium heat. Season with salt and pepper.

Per Serving:
calories: 78 | fat: 0g | protein: 3g | carbs: 15g | fiber: 3g

Kale and Lentil Stew

Prep time: 10 minutes | Cook time: 50 minutes | Serves 8

- 5 cups (2 pounds / 907 g) brown or green dry lentils
- 8 cups vegetable broth or water
- 4 cups kale, stemmed and chopped into 2-inch pieces
- 2 large carrots, diced
- 1 tablespoon smoked paprika
- 2 teaspoons onion powder
- 2 teaspoons garlic powder
- 1 teaspoon red pepper flakes
- 1 teaspoon dried oregano
- 1 teaspoon dried thyme

1. In a large stockpot, combine the lentils, broth, kale, carrots, paprika, onion powder, garlic powder, red pepper flakes, oregano, and thyme. Bring the mixture to a boil over medium-high heat. 2. Once boiling, cover the pot, reduce the heat to medium-low, and let it simmer for 45 minutes, stirring every 5 to 10 minutes to ensure even cooking. Serve the flavorful and hearty lentil soup warm and enjoy its nourishing goodness.

Per Serving:
calories: 467 | fat: 3g | protein: 32g | carbs: 78g | fiber: 31g

Kale White Bean Soup

Prep time: 20 minutes | Cook time: 2 hours | Serves 6

- 1 pound (454 g) navy beans
- 1 tablespoon coconut oil (optional)
- ½ cup coarsely chopped onions
- 1 clove garlic, minced
- ¼ cup nutritional yeast
- 1 diced red bell pepper
- 4 chopped Roma tomatoes
- 2 cups sliced carrots
- 5 cups vegetable broth
- 1 teaspoon Italian seasoning
- 2 teaspoons salt (optional)
- ½ teaspoon ground black pepper
- 1 pound (454 g) kale, de-stemmed and coarsely chopped

1. Place the beans in a large stockpot and cover with water by about 3 inches. Let it sit overnight to let the beans expand. If you want to do the quick method for preparing the beans—instead of soaking overnight—then cover beans with water by 2 inches in the stockpot. Cover with a lid and bring to a boil. Remove from the heat and let stand, uncovered, 1 hour. Drain beans in a colander and set aside. 2. Put the oil (if desired) in the same stockpot and heat over medium heat. Add the onions and sauté for about 10 to 15 minutes until soft and translucent. Add the garlic and cook, stirring, for 1 minute. Add 4 cups water, the beans, nutritional yeast, bell pepper, tomatoes, carrots, broth, Italian seasoning, salt (if desired), and pepper. Cover and bring to a boil. Uncover and turn down to a simmer. Cook until beans are tender, about 1 to 1½ hours. 3. Stir in kale and 2 cups water and simmer, uncovered, until kale is tender, about 12 to 15 minutes.

Per Serving:
calories: 131 | fat: 4g | protein: 14g | carbs: 20g | fiber: 7g

Smoky Saffron Chickpea, Chard, and Rice Soup

Prep time: 15 minutes | Cook time: 35 minutes | Serves 6

2 teaspoons virgin olive oil (optional)
1 medium yellow onion, small diced
1 stalk celery, small diced
3 cloves garlic, minced
1½ teaspoons smoked paprika
¼ cup tomato paste
1 medium zucchini, chopped into ½-inch pieces
1½ cups cooked chickpeas
⅓ cup medium-grain brown rice, rinsed
Salt and pepper, to taste (optional)
Pinch of saffron threads
5 to 6 cups vegetable stock
1 bunch chard, leaves chopped
¼ cup chopped fresh flat-leaf parsley
1 tablespoon fresh lemon juice

1. In a large soup pot, heat the olive oil over medium heat. Add the onions and celery, stirring and sautéing until the onions become soft and translucent, which takes about 5 minutes. 2. Mix in the garlic, smoked paprika, and tomato paste, stirring to combine. Add the zucchini, chickpeas, and rice. Season with salt and pepper, if desired. Add the saffron and vegetable stock, give it a good stir, and cover the pot. Bring the mixture to a boil, then reduce the heat to a gentle simmer. Cook, covered, until the rice is perfectly tender, which should take around 25 minutes. Add the chopped chard to the pot and continue cooking until it just wilts, approximately 3 minutes. 3. Finally, stir in the parsley and lemon juice, and serve the soup immediately.

Per Serving:
calories: 155 | fat: 3g | protein: 6g | carbs: 27g | fiber: 5g

Roasted Potato and Cauliflower Soup

Prep time: 20 minutes | Cook time: 30 minutes | Serves 6

8 garlic cloves, peeled
1 large cauliflower head, cut into small florets
2 russet potatoes, peeled and chopped into 1-inch pieces
1 yellow onion, coarsely chopped
1 celery stalk, coarsely chopped
1 tablespoon water, plus more as needed
6 cups no-sodium vegetable broth
2 thyme sprigs
2 teaspoons paprika
¼ teaspoon freshly ground black pepper
1 tablespoon chopped fresh rosemary leaves

1. Preheat your oven to 450ºF (235ºC) and prepare a baking sheet with parchment paper. 2. Wrap the garlic cloves in aluminum foil or place them in a garlic roaster. 3. Spread the cauliflower and potatoes evenly on the prepared baking sheet, and add the wrapped garlic cloves to the sheet. 4. Roast the vegetables for 15 to 20 minutes until the cauliflower develops a light brown color. 5. In a large 8-quart pot, set the heat to high, and combine the onion and celery. Sauté for 4 to 5 minutes, adding water as needed, one tablespoon at a time, to prevent burning and help the onion to brown slightly. 6. Pour in the vegetable broth and bring the soup to a gentle simmer. 7. Add the roasted vegetables, including the garlic, along with thyme, paprika, and pepper. Allow the soup to simmer, covering the pot, for approximately 10 minutes. 8. Remove the thyme sprigs and discard. Use an immersion blender to puree the soup until it becomes smooth. If you find the consistency too thick, add water as required until it reaches your desired thickness. Stir in the rosemary to complete the soup.

Per Serving:
calories: 120 | fat: 1g | protein: 5g | carbs: 26g | fiber: 5g

Broccoli and "Cheddar" Soup

Prep time: 10 minutes | Cook time: 30 minutes | Serves 4

4 cups peeled and diced butternut squash
2 sweet potatoes, peeled and diced (about 2 cups)
1 small yellow onion, peeled and halved
2 garlic cloves, peeled
4 cups water
2 teaspoons salt (optional)
1 (13-ounce / 369-g) can light unsweetened coconut milk
1 tablespoon red miso paste
3 tablespoons nutritional yeast
1 tablespoon tapioca flour
3 cups frozen broccoli

1. In a large pot, combine the butternut squash, sweet potatoes, onion, garlic, and water and bring to a boil over high heat. Lower the heat to medium-low and cook until fork-tender, about 20 minutes. 2. Transfer the mixture (including the liquid) to a blender and purée until smooth. You may need to do this in batches. 3. Return the soup to the pot and add the salt (if using), coconut milk, red miso, nutritional yeast, tapioca flour, and broccoli and cook over medium heat, stirring often, until heated through, about 10 minutes.

Per Serving:
calories: 353 | fat: 20g | protein: 8g | carbs: 42g | fiber: 9g

Lime-Mint Soup

Prep time: 5 minutes | Cook time: 20 minutes | Serves 4

4 cups vegetable broth
¼ cup fresh mint leaves, roughly chopped
¼ cup chopped scallions, white and green parts
3 minced garlic cloves
3 tablespoons freshly squeezed lime juice

1. In a large stockpot, combine the broth, mint, scallions, garlic, and lime juice. Bring to a boil over medium-high heat. 2. Cover, reduce the heat to low, simmer for 15 minutes, and serve.

Per Serving:
calories: 55 | fat: 2g | protein: 5g | carbs: 5g | fiber: 1g

Split Pea Soup

Prep time: 15 minutes | Cook time: 1 hour | Serves 4

2 cups dried split peas
1 (7-ounce / 198-g) pack smoked tofu, cubed
5 cups vegetable stock
2 small onions, minced

4 carrots, sliced
Optional Toppings:
Parsley
Black pepper
Nigella seeds

1. Begin by placing a large pot over medium-high heat and adding the vegetable stock and split peas. 2. Bring the stock to a boil and then reduce the heat to medium.
3. Allow the split peas to cook uncovered for approximately 40 minutes. 4. While cooking, skim off any foam that may develop and stir the peas occasionally.
5. Next, add the smoked tofu cubes, carrots, and onions to the pot. Lower the heat to a simmer, cover the pot with a lid, and let it simmer for an additional 20 minutes, stirring occasionally. 6. Turn off the heat and allow the soup to cool down for 5 minutes.
7. Divide the soup into two bowls, serve with optional toppings, and enjoy!
8. If there are leftovers, store the soup in an airtight container in the fridge and consume within 2 days. Alternatively, you can store it in the freezer for up to 60 days. When reheating, either use a pot or the microwave.

Per Serving:
calories: 176 | fat: 4g | protein: 21g | carbs: 14g | fiber: 17g

Lentil Chili

Prep time: 30 minutes | Cook time: 55 minutes | Serves 6 to 8

3 medium yellow onions, peeled and chopped (about 1½ cups)
1½ cups chopped celery
2 medium carrots, peeled and sliced (about 1 cup)
2 medium bell peppers, seeded and chopped (about 1 cup)
1 to 2 cloves garlic, peeled and minced
6 cups vegetable stock, or low-sodium vegetable broth
1½ tablespoons chili powder
1 teaspoon ground cumin

1 teaspoon paprika
½ teaspoon chipotle powder or smoked paprika
½ teaspoon cayenne pepper
2 cups red lentils, rinsed
1 (28-ounce / 794-g) can crushed tomatoes
1 (15-ounce / 425-g) can kidney beans, drained and rinsed
Zest and juice of 1 lime
Salt and freshly ground black pepper, to taste

1. Place the onion, celery, carrots, bell peppers, garlic, and 1 cup of the vegetable stock in a large pot over medium-high heat. Cook, stirring occasionally, until the vegetables soften, 5 to 7 minutes. Add the chili powder, cumin, paprika, chipotle powder, and cayenne pepper and cook for an additional minute, stirring well. 2. Add the lentils, tomatoes, kidney beans, and the remaining vegetable stock to the pot. Cover and bring to a boil over high heat. Reduce the heat to medium-low and simmer, stirring occasionally, until the lentils are soft, about 45 minutes. Add the lime zest and juice and season with salt and pepper.

Per Serving:
calories: 279 | fat: 1g | protein: 16g | carbs: 52g | fiber: 11g

Leaf and Stem Green Tortilla Soup

Prep time: 15 minutes | Cook time: 35 minutes | Serves 5

¾ pound (340 g) fresh tomatillos, papery skins removed
8 small corn tortillas
2 tablespoons coconut oil, divided
1 medium white onion, chopped
4 cloves garlic, chopped
1 jalapeño pepper, deseeded and chopped
2 teaspoons ground cumin

2 teaspoons ground coriander
5 cups vegetable stock
3 cups chopped greens with stems
Salt and pepper, to taste (optional)
Serve:
Tortilla strips
Diced ripe avocado
Chopped fresh cilantro leaves
Lime wedges

1. Place the top oven rack about 3 to 4 inches from the broiler. Preheat the broiler to high. Place the peeled tomatillos on a baking sheet and slide the baking sheet into the oven. Broil the tomatillos for 8 to 10 minutes or until lightly blackened and slightly oozing. Set the broiled tomatillos aside to cool. 2. Lower the oven temperature to 400°F (205°C). Cut the tortillas into strips and lay them on a baking sheet. Toss the tortilla strips with 1 tablespoon of the coconut oil and some salt, if using. After the strips are evenly coated, arrange them in a single layer, and slide the baking sheet into the oven. Bake until the tortilla strips are lightly browned and crisp, about 15 minutes. Remove from oven and set aside. 3. Heat the remaining 1 tablespoon of the coconut oil in a large pot over medium heat. Add the white onions to the pot and sauté until soft and translucent, about 4 minutes. Add the garlic, jalapeño, cumin, and coriander. Stir for about 30 seconds or until the garlic is very fragrant. 4. Add the broiled tomatillos and vegetable stock to the pot. Bring to a boil. Add ⅓ of the baked tortilla strips and all the chopped greens and their stems. Cook until the greens are vibrant green, about 1 minute. Remove from the heat. 5. With a blender, purée the soup in batches until totally smooth. Once all the soup is puréed, return it to the pot and bring it back to a boil on the stove. Season the soup with salt and pepper. 6. Serve the soup hot and garnished with the remaining baked tortilla strips, diced avocado, chopped cilantro, and lime wedges on the side.

Per Serving: (1 cup)
calories: 239 | fat: 8g | protein: 7g | carbs: 54g | fiber: 9g

Bean and Mushroom Chili

Prep time: 20 minutes | Cook time: 38 minutes | Serves 6

1 large onion, peeled and chopped
1 pound (454 g) button mushrooms, chopped
6 cloves garlic, peeled and minced
1 tablespoon ground cumin
1 tablespoon ancho chile powder
4 teaspoons ground fennel
½ teaspoon cayenne pepper, or to taste
1 tablespoon unsweetened cocoa powder
1 (28-ounce / 794-g) can diced tomatoes
4 cups cooked pinto beans, or 2 (15-ounce / 425-g) cans, drained and rinsed
Salt, to taste (optional)

1. Place the onion and mushrooms in a large saucepan and sauté over medium heat for 10 minutes. Add water 1 to 2 tablespoons at a time to keep the vegetables from sticking to the pan. 2. Add the garlic, cumin, chile powder, fennel, cayenne pepper, and cocoa powder and cook for 3 minutes. Add the tomatoes, beans, and 2 cups of water and simmer, covered, for 25 minutes. Season with salt, if using.

Per Serving:
calories: 229 | fat: 1g | protein: 14g | carbs: 42g | fiber: 15g

Brown Lentil Stew with Avocado Salsa

Prep time: 15 minutes | Cook time: 40 minutes | Serves 4

Stew:
1 cup brown lentils, rinsed
½ teaspoon salt, or to taste (optional)
½ teaspoon turmeric
1 medium green bell pepper, seeded and chopped (about ½ cup)
½ cup chopped celery
½ cup chopped tomato
½ teaspoon curry powder
½ teaspoon fresh lime juice
Avocado Salsa:
½ avocado, halved, pitted, peeled and cut into ½-inch cubes (about ½ cup)
½ cup finely diced tomato
½ teaspoon finely chopped cilantro
½ teaspoon fresh lime juice
¼ teaspoon freshly ground black pepper

Make the Stew: 1. Place the lentils, salt (if using), turmeric, and 2 cups of water in a large saucepan. Cook, uncovered, over medium heat for 25 to 30 minutes. Add the green pepper, celery, tomato, and curry powder and cook for 10 minutes. Just before serving, add the lime juice. Make the Avocado Salsa: 2. Combine the avocado, tomato, cilantro, lime juice, and black pepper in a medium bowl. Mix well to combine. 3. Serve the stew hot and top with the avocado salsa.

Per Serving:
calories: 226 | fat: 4g | protein: 13g | carbs: 36g | fiber: 8g

Chapter 10: Staples, Sauces, Dips, and Dressings

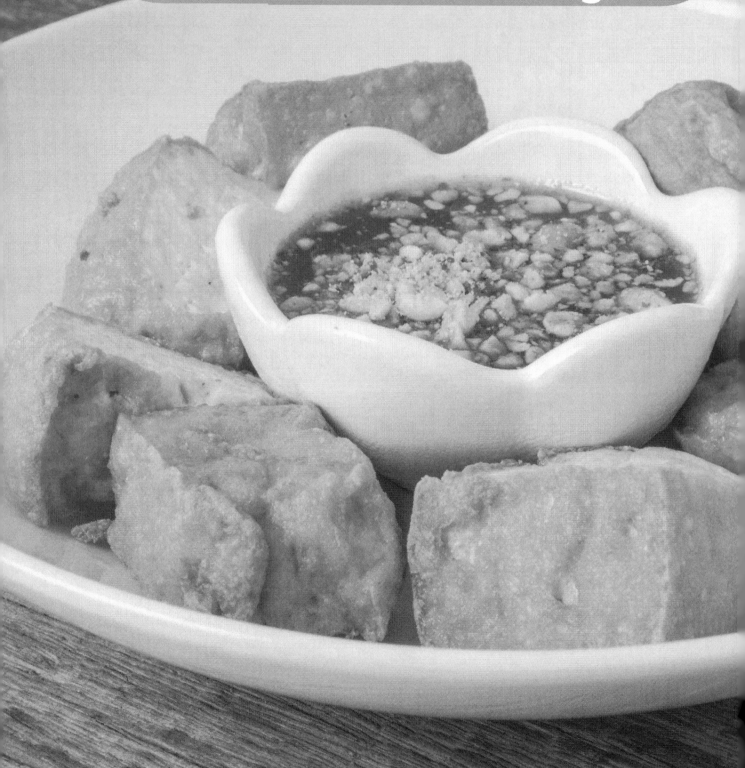

Nut or Seed Butter

Prep time: 5 minutes | Cook time: 0 minutes | Makes 1 cup

2 cups raw whole nuts or seeds, toasted

1 teaspoon flaky sea salt, or to taste (optional)

1. Place the nuts or seeds in a food processor and process for approximately 2 minutes, or until they clump together to form a ball. Break up the ball, scrape down the sides of the processor, and continue blending for an additional 3 to 4 minutes, or until the butter becomes smooth and liquid. Scrape the sides of the processor once more, then add the flaky salt and pulse to combine. Store the resulting mixture in a sealed glass jar or an airtight container at room temperature for up to 1 month. If the weather is hot, it's advisable to store it in the fridge.

Per Serving: (⅛ cup)

calories: 207 | fat: 18g | protein: 8g | carbs: 8g | fiber: 2g

Cauliflower Bake Topping

Prep time: 10 minutes | Cook time: 15 minutes | Serves 6

1 large head cauliflower, cut into 1½-inch florets
½ cup raw pine nuts, cashews, or macadamia nuts
½ cup filtered water if using a food processor
2 tablespoons extra-virgin olive oil (optional)
3 tablespoons nutritional yeast, plus more to taste
½ teaspoon fine sea salt, plus more to taste (optional)

1. Prepare a steamer pot with about 2 inches of filtered water in the bottom, ensuring that the water level doesn't touch the steamer basket. Bring the water to a boil over high heat. Place the cauliflower florets in the steamer basket, cover, and steam for 10 to 12 minutes until the cauliflower is cooked through but still firm. Remove from heat and set aside. 2. High-Powered-Blender Method: In a high-powered blender, combine the nuts, olive oil, nutritional yeast, and optional salt. Add the steamed cauliflower to the blender. Start on low speed and use the tamper stick to press the cauliflower down, gradually increasing the speed to high. Blend until the mixture becomes completely smooth and thick. Use the tamper stick to keep the mixture moving and scrape down the sides as needed. This process will take a couple of minutes. Season with more nutritional yeast and salt according to taste, and blend to combine. 3. Food-Processor Method: Place the steamed cauliflower in a food processor. In a regular upright blender, blend the nuts, water, olive oil, nutritional yeast, and salt until smooth. Pour this mixture into the food processor with the cauliflower. Process until the mixture becomes completely smooth, occasionally scraping down the sides as necessary. Add more nutritional yeast and salt to taste. 4. The topping is now ready to be baked on a filling of your choice, or you can store it in an airtight container in the fridge for up to 3 days, or freeze it for up to 3 months.

Per Serving:

calories: 167 | fat: 13g | protein: 6g | carbs: 10g | fiber: 4g

Creamy Nut Sauce

Prep time: 15 minutes | Cook time: 20 minutes | Makes 2 cups

1 tablespoon extra-virgin coconut oil (optional)
1 medium onion, diced
3 large garlic cloves, finely chopped
½ teaspoon fine sea salt, plus more to taste (optional)
1 tablespoon mirin
¼ cup filtered water
1 cup raw or toasted cashews, walnuts, or almonds
¾ cup boiling filtered water
1 teaspoon tamari

1. Heat the oil in a medium skillet over medium-high heat. Add the onion and sauté until it turns golden, which should take around 6 to 8 minutes. Stir in the garlic and salt (if using), and cook for an additional 3 to 4 minutes until the garlic becomes fragrant and also turns golden. Pour in the mirin and ¼ cup of water, then increase the heat and bring the mixture to a simmer. Stir the contents for a couple of minutes to deglaze the pan. 2. Remove the skillet from the heat and transfer the cooked mixture to an upright blender, ensuring to scrape all the contents from the skillet using a rubber spatula. Add the nuts, boiling water, and tamari to the blender and blend everything until it becomes smooth, occasionally scraping down the sides of the blender as needed. Taste the mixture and season with more salt if desired. You can serve it immediately, or if you prefer, let it cool down and store it in an airtight jar in the refrigerator for up to 4 days.

Per Serving: (½ cup)

calories: 188 | fat: 16g | protein: 4g | carbs: 9g | fiber: 2g

Oil-Free Sundried Tomato and Oregano Dressing

Prep time: 10 minutes | Cook time: 5 minutes | Makes 3 cups

2 cups filtered water
½ cup sundried tomato halves
1 clove garlic, chopped
1 small shallot, chopped
2 tablespoons Dijon mustard
2 tablespoons pure maple syrup (optional)
¼ teaspoon dried oregano
salt and pepper, to taste (optional)

1. Boil 2 cups of water. In a small bowl, combine the sundried tomatoes with the boiling water and allow them to soften for approximately 10 minutes. 2. Transfer the softened sundried tomatoes along with the soaking liquid to a blender. Add the garlic, shallots, Dijon mustard, maple syrup, oregano, and optional salt and pepper. Blend the mixture on high speed until it turns smooth and creamy. This process typically takes about 3 minutes, with a few pauses to scrape down the sides of the blender. Store the dressing in the refrigerator for up to 1 week.

Per Serving: (½ cup)

calories: 37 | fat: 0g | protein: 1g | carbs: 8g | fiber: 1g

Spring All-Purpose Seasoning

Prep time: 5 minutes | Cook time: 0 minutes | Makes ½ cup

3 tablespoons dried dill
3 tablespoons dried thyme
2 tablespoons dried tarragon

1. In a jar with a tight-fitting lid, shake all the ingredients. Store for up to 6 months.

Per Serving: (½ cup)
calories: 93 | fat: 4g | protein: 5g | carbs: 18g | fiber: 7g

Mild Harissa Sauce

Prep time: 10 minutes | Cook time: 20 minutes | Makes 3 to 4 cups

1 large red bell pepper, seeded, cored, and cut into chunks
1 yellow onion, cut into thick rings
4 garlic cloves, peeled
1 cup no-sodium vegetable broth or water
2 tablespoons tomato paste
1 tablespoon low-sodium soy sauce or tamari
1 tablespoon Hungarian paprika
1 teaspoon ground cumin

1. Preheat your oven to 450ºF (235ºC) and line a baking sheet with parchment paper or aluminum foil. 2. Place the bell pepper on the prepared baking sheet with the flesh-side facing up. Arrange the onion and garlic around the pepper. 3. Roast the vegetables on the middle rack of the oven for 20 minutes. Once done, transfer them to a blender. 4. Add the vegetable broth, tomato paste, soy sauce, paprika, and cumin to the blender with the roasted vegetables. Blend the mixture until it becomes smooth. This flavorful sauce can be served either cold or warm. 5. For storage, you can refrigerate the sauce in an airtight container for up to 2 weeks, or if you prefer, freeze it for up to 6 months.

Per Serving: (¼ cup)
calories: 15 | fat: 0g | protein: 1g | carbs: 3g | fiber: 1g

Lemon Mint Tahini Cream

Prep time: 5 minutes | Cook time: 0 minutes | Serves 6

½ cup tahini
3 pitted dates
½ cup water
¼ cup lemon juice
2 cloves garlic
6 leaves mint

1. Place all the ingredients in a blender or food processor and blend until a thick and smooth sauce is formed. 2. Store the tahini cream in the refrigerator using an airtight container and consume it within 3 days. Alternatively, you can freeze the tahini cream for up to 60 days and thaw it at room temperature when needed.

Per Serving:
calories: 141 | fat: 11g | protein: 5g | carbs: 5g | fiber: 1g

Creamy Balsamic Dressing

Prep time: 10 minutes | Cook time: 0 minutes | Makes ¾ cup

¼ cup tahini
¼ cup balsamic vinegar
¼ cup fresh basil, minced
⅛ cup water
1 tablespoon maple syrup
(optional)
1 garlic clove, pressed
Pinch sea salt (optional)
Pinch freshly ground black pepper (optional)

1. In a blender or food processor, put all the ingredients and blend until smooth. You could whisk this together without a blender, if you mince the basil very fine.

Per Serving: (1 tablespoon)
calories: 157 | fat: 10g | protein: 3g | carbs: 12g | fiber: 2g

Kalamata Olives and White Bean Dip

Prep time: 5 minutes | Cook time: 0 minutes | Makes 1 cup

5 jumbo Kalamata olives, pitted
1 cup cooked cannellini beans (no added salt)
1 tablespoon tahini (no added sugar or salt)
1 garlic clove
1 tablespoon freshly squeezed lemon juice
1 tablespoon water

1. In a food processor, mix the olives, beans, tahini, garlic, lemon juice, and water and blend until it reaches the desired consistency.

Per Serving:
calories: 95 | fat: 3g | protein: 5g | carbs: 13g | fiber: 4g

Peanut Butter Apple Sauce

Prep time: 10 minutes | Cook time: 15 minutes | Serves 16

4 large apples, peeled and cored
½ cup peanut butter
¼ cup raisins
1 tablespoon cinnamon
½ cup water

1. Cut the cored and peeled apples into tiny pieces and add them to the saucepan. 2. Add the water to the saucepan and put it over low heat, then cover the saucepan with a lid and bring it to a boil. 3. Cook the apples for about 15 minutes or until they are soft, then turn off the heat and mash the apples with a fork or a potato masher. 4. Add the peanut butter and stir thoroughly until everything is well combined. 5. Add more water if the sauce is too thick, then add the raisins and cinnamon. 6. Stir again until everything is mixed thoroughly, serve warm or cold and enjoy! 7. Store the sauce in the fridge, using an airtight container, and consume within 3 days. Store the sauce in the freezer for a maximum of 60 days and thaw at room temperature.

Per Serving:
calories: 91 | fat: 4g | protein: 2g | carbs: 12g | fiber: 2g

Refrigerator Pickles

Prep time: 20 minutes | Cook time: 10 minutes | Makes 2 pints

1 pound (454 g) small cucumbers, preferably pickling cucumbers, washed and dried
1 small yellow onion, chopped or cut into rings
1 cup apple cider vinegar
1 cup water
¼ cup beet sugar (optional)
1 tablespoon kosher salt (optional)
1 tablespoon pickling spice

1. Slice the unpeeled cucumbers into ¼-inch-thick rounds using a sharp knife or mandoline. 2. In a large bowl, combine the cucumbers and onions thoroughly. Split the mixture evenly between two 1-pint wide-mouth canning jars, leaving about ½ inch of space from the top where the lids will seal. Gently pack the vegetables using a clean hand or a sturdy spoon, being cautious not to break the cucumbers. 3. In a small pot over high heat, combine the vinegar, water, beet sugar, and pickling spice. Stir and bring the mixture to a boil until the sugar and salt (if using) dissolve completely. Pour the brine over the vegetables, leaving ½ inch of space from the top. You might not need all the brine. Loosely close the lids and lightly tap the jars on the counter to release any air bubbles. If necessary, add more brine to reach the ½-inch line before sealing the jars tightly. Allow the jars to cool to room temperature.
4. Refrigerate the jars for at least 24 hours before serving. As time passes, the pickles will develop even more flavor and maintain a crisp texture compared to store-bought ones. 5. Due to the high acidity of the brine, you can keep these pickles refrigerated for 1 month or more. However, since they haven't gone through a canning process, they are not shelf-stable.

Per Serving: (4 pickles)
calories: 218 | fat: 1g | protein: 4g | carbs: 50g | fiber: 7g

Smoky Mushrooms

Prep time: 10 minutes | Cook time: 10 minutes | Makes 2 cups

2 tablespoons soy sauce
2 tablespoons pure maple syrup
1 tablespoon liquid smoke
1 tablespoon liquid aminos
¼ teaspoon freshly ground black pepper
1 pound (454 g) cremini mushrooms, cut into ½-inch-thick slices

1. In a sauté pan or skillet, combine the soy sauce, maple syrup, liquid smoke, liquid aminos, and pepper, whisking them together. 2. Add the mushrooms to the mixture and cook over medium-high heat, stirring frequently, for approximately 10 minutes. The liquid should evaporate, leaving the mushrooms tender and glossy. Once done, remove the pan from the heat. Store the cooked mushrooms in an airtight container in the refrigerator until you're ready to use them.

Per Serving:
calories: 45 | fat: 0g | protein: 3g | carbs: 8g | fiber: 1g

Korean Tahini BBQ Sauce

Prep time: 10 minutes | Cook time: 0 minutes | Makes ¾ cup

½ cup water
¼ cup red miso
1 piece ginger, peeled and minced
3 cloves garlic, minced
2 tablespoons chili paste or chili sauce
2 tablespoons rice vinegar
2 tablespoons tahini

1. In a mini blender, purée all the ingredients until smooth. Serve as is or thin with an additional ½ cup water and use as a marinade for tofu, tempeh, or portobello mushroom caps.

Per Serving: (¼ cup)
calories: 124 | fat: 7g | protein: 5g | carbs: 12g | fiber: 3g

Cilantro-Coconut Pesto

Prep time: 5 minutes | Cook time: 0 minutes | Serves 8

1 (13½-ounce / 383-g) can full-fat coconut milk
1 bunch cilantro leaves
2 jalapeños
1 piece ginger, peeled and minced
1 tablespoon white miso
Water, as needed

1. In a blender, process the coconut milk, cilantro, jalapeños, ginger, and miso until smooth. Thin with water as needed. The pesto can be refrigerated for up to 2 days, or divided into resealable containers and frozen for up to 6 months.

Per Serving:
calories: 122 | fat: 12g | protein: 2g | carbs: 4g | fiber: 1g

Veggie Chow Mein

Prep time: 10 minutes | Cook time: 15 minutes | Serves 6

1 (8-ounce / 227-g) package Asian-style noodles
3 tablespoons water
1 cup thinly sliced celery
½ cup diced red, white, or yellow onion
½ cup grated carrots
1 teaspoon minced garlic
½ cup vegetable broth
2 tablespoons soy sauce
1 cup bean sprouts

1. In a large pot over medium-high heat, boil water and cook the noodles according to the directions on the package. 2. While the noodles are cooking, prepare the vegetables. In a large pan or wok, heat the water. Add the celery, onion, carrots, and garlic and sauté for 3 to 4 minutes or until the celery and onion are tender and the onion is translucent. 3. Add the broth and soy sauce. Bring to a boil, then turn down the heat and simmer for 5 minutes. 4. Add the cooked noodles and bean sprouts and mix thoroughly. Cook for 5 minutes, stirring occasionally.

Per Serving:
calories: 86 | fat: 1g | protein: 4g | carbs: 16g | fiber: 1g

Sour Cream

Prep time: 5 minutes | **Cook time:** 0 minutes | Serves 10

- 1 cup coconut cream
- 2 tablespoons lemon juice
- ½ teaspoon apple cider vinegar
- ½ teaspoon salt (optional)

1. To make the sour cream, combine all the ingredients in a food processor or blender and blend until you achieve a smooth consistency. Alternatively, you can place all the ingredients in a medium bowl and use hand mixers to whisk until smooth. 2. Chill the sour cream before serving and savor it as a delightful topping or side dish! 3. For storage, keep the sour cream in the refrigerator using an airtight container and consume it within 4 days. Alternatively, you can store it in the freezer for up to 60 days, and when needed, thaw it at room temperature.

Per Serving:
calories: 20 | fat: 1g | protein: 0g | carbs: 3g | fiber: 0g

Perfect Marinara Sauce

Prep time: 10 minutes | **Cook time:** 20 minutes | Makes 7 cups

- 2 (28-ounce / 794-g) cans crushed tomatoes in purée
- 4 garlic cloves, minced
- 2 tablespoons Italian seasoning
- 2 teaspoons pure maple syrup
- 2 teaspoons onion powder
- 2 teaspoons paprika
- ¼ teaspoon freshly ground black pepper

1. Combine the tomatoes, garlic, Italian seasoning, maple syrup, onion powder, paprika, and pepper in a medium saucepan. Bring the mixture to a simmer. 2. Once simmering, lower the heat to a gentle setting. Cover the saucepan and let it simmer for 15 to 20 minutes, allowing the sauce to become fragrant and the flavors to blend harmoniously. When ready, remove the saucepan from the heat.

Per Serving:
calories: 39 | fat: 0g | protein: 2g | carbs: 8g | fiber: 2g

Plant-Powered "Sour Cream"

Prep time: 5 minutes | **Cook time:** 0 minutes | Makes 1 cup

- 8 ounces (227 g) silken tofu
- 2 tablespoons freshly squeezed lemon juice
- 1 teaspoon apple cider vinegar
- 1 teaspoon onion powder

1. Mix the tofu, lemon juice, vinegar, and onion powder in a blender. Blend for 1 minute, or until the mixture reaches a creamy consistency. 2. Store in a refrigerator-safe container for up to 5 days.

Per Serving: (1 tablespoon)
calories: 10 | fat: 0g | protein: 1g | carbs: 0g | fiber: 0g

Whipped Lentil Chipotle Dip

Prep time: 10 minutes | **Cook time:** 10 minutes | Makes 2 cups

- 1 cup split red lentils, rinsed
- 3 cloves garlic, peeled
- 2 chipotle peppers in adobo
- 1 tablespoon adobo sauce from the can (optional)
- 3 tablespoons raw cashew butter
- 1 tablespoon fresh lemon juice
- 1 teaspoon tomato paste
- 1½ teaspoons ground cumin
- Salt and pepper, to taste (optional)
- Garnishes (optional):
- Virgin olive oil (optional)
- Ground cumin
- Sweet paprika

1. Place the lentils in a medium saucepan and cover them with 3 cups of filtered water. Bring to a boil over medium-high heat. Lower to a simmer and cook until the lentils are mushy and falling apart, about 8 minutes. 2. While the lentils are cooking, combine the garlic, chipotles, adobo, if using, cashew butter, lemon juice, tomato paste, and cumin in a blender. 3. Drain the cooked lentils, and scrape them into the blender with the garlic and chipotle mixture. Season with salt and pepper, if using. Whiz everything on high until the dip is completely smooth. You may have to stop the blender and scrape down the sides a couple of times. 4. The dip will be quite warm. For optimal serving, scrape the dip into a container and cover it with plastic wrap, pressing it onto the surface of the dip. Refrigerate the dip for at least 1 hour before serving. 5. You can garnish the top with a drizzle of olive oil, some extra ground cumin, and a sprinkle of paprika if you like.

Per Serving: (½ cup)
calories: 261 | fat: 7g | protein: 14g | carbs: 38g | fiber: 6g

Basil Pesto

Prep time: 10 minutes | **Cook time:** 0 minutes | Makes about 1½ cups

- 1 cup fresh basil, chopped
- ½ cup pine nuts, or walnuts, or sunflower seeds
- 1 to 2 garlic cloves, pressed
- Zest and juice of 1 small lemon
- 2 tablespoons nutritional yeast (optional)
- ¼ cup avocado, or 2 tablespoons tahini (optional)
- ⅛ teaspoon sea salt (optional)

1. For the sweetest flavor from fresh basil, immerse the leaves in a large bowl of ice water and let them soak for approximately 5 minutes before chopping. 2. To enhance the flavor, you have the option to lightly toast the nuts. Place them in a small skillet on medium heat, stirring frequently. Alternatively, you can toast them in the oven at 300°F (150°C) for 8 to 10 minutes. Keep a close eye on them, as small nuts and seeds can burn quickly. If you prefer, you can skip this step and proceed directly to step 3. 3. In a food processor or blender, blend all the ingredients until a smooth consistency is achieved. Taste the mixture and add more salt (if using) or other seasonings as needed.

Per Serving: (1 tablespoon)
calories: 89 | fat: 8g | protein: 1g | carbs: 2g | fiber: 0g

Quick Mole Sauce

Prep time: 40 minutes | Cook time: 25 minutes | Makes 4 cups

4 dried pasilla chiles
2 dried ancho chiles
Boiling water, for soaking the peppers
1 yellow onion, cut into slices
6 garlic cloves, coarsely chopped
1 tablespoon water, plus more as needed
2 tablespoons tomato paste
1 jalapeño pepper, seeded and chopped
2 ounces (57 g) vegan dark chocolate
2 tablespoons whole wheat flour
2 tablespoons cocoa powder
2 tablespoons almond butter
2 teaspoons smoked paprika
1 teaspoon ground cumin
1 teaspoon ground cinnamon
½ teaspoon dried oregano
2½ cups no-sodium vegetable broth

1. Remove the stem ends from the pasilla and ancho chiles, and shake out the seeds. Cut the chiles in half, then transfer them to a medium bowl and cover with boiling water. Let them soak for 20 minutes, and then drain. 2. In a large nonstick sauté pan or skillet over medium-high heat, combine the onion and garlic. Cook for 5 to 7 minutes, adding water 1 tablespoon at a time to prevent burning. The onions should turn dark brown without getting burnt. Stir in the tomato paste and cook for an additional 2 minutes to caramelize. Transfer this mixture to a high-speed blender.
3. Add the soaked chiles, jalapeño pepper, chocolate, flour, cocoa powder, almond butter, paprika, cumin, cinnamon, oregano, and vegetable broth to the blender. Purée the ingredients for about 3 minutes until a smooth sauce is formed.
4. Return the sauté pan or skillet to medium-high heat. Pour in the sauce and cover the pan. Cook until the sauce begins to bubble. Then, reduce the heat to low and let it simmer uncovered for 5 minutes, stirring occasionally. 5. The sauce is now ready to be served immediately. You can also refrigerate it in an airtight container for up to 1 week or freeze it for up to 6 months.

Per Serving: (½ cup)
calories: 114 | fat: 7g | protein: 4g | carbs: 13g | fiber: 4g

Spaghetti Squash with Marinara and Veggies

Prep time: 15 minutes | Cook time: 10 minutes | Serves 4

3 tablespoons water
½ green or red bell pepper, diced
½ cup diced red, white, or yellow onion
1 teaspoon minced garlic
2 cups chopped spinach
1 (14½-ounce / 411-g) can diced tomatoes with their juices
½ tablespoon dried oregano
1 (15-ounce / 425-g) can black or pinto beans, drained and rinsed
¼ teaspoon salt (optional)
1 roasted spaghetti squash, cut in half

1. Heat water in a large pan over medium-high heat. Add the bell pepper, onion, and garlic, and sauté for about 3 minutes, until the onion turns tender and translucent.
2. Stir in the spinach, tomatoes, oregano, beans, and optional salt. Reduce the heat to low and let the mixture simmer for 5 minutes. 3. As the vegetables cook, use a fork to scrape the inside of the roasted spaghetti squash, creating spaghetti-like strands.
4. Finally, pour the pepper and tomato sauce over the spaghetti squash.

Per Serving:
calories: 153 | fat: 1g | protein: 7g | carbs: 32g | fiber: 8g

Pico de Gallo

Prep time: 15 minutes | Cook time: 0 minutes | Makes 2 cups

4 tomatoes, chopped small
1 medium yellow onion, minced
1 jalapeño pepper, seeded and minced
Juice of 1 lime, plus more if needed
Pinch of salt, plus more if needed (optional)
3 tablespoons chopped fresh cilantro

1. Combine the tomatoes, onion, jalapeño, lime juice, salt (if using), and cilantro in a large bowl. Taste and adjust seasoning if desired. The salsa can be stored in an airtight container in the refrigerator for up to 4 days.

Per Serving:
calories: 19 | fat: 0g | protein: 1g | carbs: 4g | fiber: 1g

Quick Spelt Bread

Prep time: 5 minutes | Cook time: 45 minutes | Makes 1 loaf

420 grams whole-grain spelt flour (about 3¾ cups)
1 teaspoon baking soda
1 teaspoon baking powder
1½ cups unsweetened soy milk
2 tablespoons pure maple syrup
1 tablespoon lemon juice

1. Preheat the oven to 350ºF (180ºC). 2. Cut parchment paper to evenly line a 9-by-5-inch loaf pan by cutting inward to make the corners fit snugly. Allow the parchment paper to pass the top of the loaf pan (you will use these to remove the loaf from the pan in step 7). 3. In a large bowl, mix together the flour, baking soda, and baking powder. 4. In a medium bowl, mix together the soy milk, maple syrup, and lemon juice. 5. Add the soy milk mixture to the flour mixture, and mix well until combined, all the flour has hydrated, gluten has started to form, and the dough gets a little harder to mix. Transfer to the prepared loaf pan. 6. Bake for 45 minutes, or until the loaf is golden brown and a wooden skewer inserted into the center comes out clean. Remove from the oven. 7. Using the parchment paper as a sling, remove the bread from the loaf pan, and let cool completely before cutting.

Per Serving:
calories: 204 | fat: 2g | protein: 8g | carbs: 42g | fiber: 6g

Creamy Mushroom Gravy

Prep time: 10 minutes | Cook time: 15 minutes | Makes 3 cups

- 8 ounces (227 g) baby portabella mushrooms, diced
- 4 ounces (113 g) shiitake mushrooms, stemmed and diced
- 1 small yellow onion, diced
- 1 garlic clove, minced
- 1 tablespoon water, plus more as needed
- 3 tablespoons whole wheat flour
- 2 tablespoons tamari or coconut aminos
- ½ teaspoon freshly ground black pepper
- ¼ teaspoon ground white pepper
- 2 cups oat milk

1. Heat a large sauté pan or skillet over medium-high heat. Cook the portabella and shiitake mushrooms for 3 to 5 minutes until all the moisture evaporates and the edges of the mushrooms start to blacken. Add the onion and garlic, and cook for an additional 5 minutes. To prevent burning, add water 1 tablespoon at a time. The onion should turn browned. 2. Stir in the flour, tamari, black pepper, and white pepper, ensuring the cooked vegetables are well coated and combined. 3. Pour in the milk and cook, whisking, until the gravy bubbles. Reduce the heat to low and continue cooking for 5 minutes, whisking occasionally, until the gravy thickens.
4. Serve the gravy fresh or reheat it as needed. You can store it in a sealed glass container in the refrigerator for up to 1 week or freeze it for up to 4 months. It's advisable to use glass containers for freezing liquids to avoid any metallic taste that may be caused by metal containers.

Per Serving: (½ cup)
calories: 81 | fat: 1g | protein: 4g | carbs: 15g | fiber: 3g

Quick Bean Sauce

Prep time: 15 minutes | Cook time: 30 minutes | Makes 3 cups

- 2 tablespoons extra-virgin coconut or olive oil (optional)
- 1 medium onion, diced
- ½ teaspoon fine sea salt, plus more to taste (optional)
- 3 large garlic cloves, finely chopped
- 2 teaspoons chopped fresh thyme
- 2 (15½-ounce / 439-g) cans black beans, drained and rinsed well
- 1 cup filtered water
- 2 teaspoons raw apple cider vinegar

1. Warm the oil in a large skillet over medium-high heat. Add the onion and salt, if using, and cook for 5 minutes, or until the onion is light golden. Cover the pan, reduce the heat to low, and cook the onion for another 5 minutes, or until soft and beginning to brown. Stir in the garlic and cook, uncovered, for 3 to 4 minutes, until fragrant. Add the thyme and cook for 2 minutes. Stir in the beans and the water, raise the heat, and bring the mixture to a boil, then cover the pan, reduce the heat to low, and simmer for 5 minutes. Remove the lid and cook for another 5 minutes, or until the mixture is creamy and the beans are very soft. (If you would like a thicker sauce, continue cooking, uncovered, until the sauce reaches the desired consistency.) You can crush some of the beans with the back of a spoon to create a creamier, smoother sauce if you like. Stir in the vinegar and season with more salt to taste. 2. Serve immediately, or let cool and store in an airtight container in the fridge for up to 4 days.

Per Serving: (½ cup)
calories: 299 | fat: 6g | protein: 16g | carbs: 48g | fiber: 12g

Harissa

Prep time: 5 minutes | Cook time: 0 minutes | Makes ½ cup

- 2 tablespoons caraway seeds
- 2 tablespoons coriander seeds
- 2 tablespoons cumin seeds
- 2 teaspoons dried mint
- 2 teaspoons garlic powder
- 1 teaspoon sweet paprika
- 1 teaspoon crushed red pepper (optional)

1. Use a clean coffee grinder to grind the caraway, coriander, and cumin. Once ground, transfer the spices to a jar with a secure lid. Add the mint, garlic powder, paprika, and optional crushed red pepper to the jar. Shake the jar vigorously to combine all the ingredients. The spice blend can be stored for up to 6 months.

Per Serving: (⅓ cup)
calories: 150 | fat: 7g | protein: 8g | carbs: 24g | fiber: 12g

Coconut "Bacon" Bits

Prep time: 15 minutes | Cook time: 12 minutes | Makes 2 cups

- 2 tablespoons tamari or low-sodium soy sauce
- 1 tablespoon liquid hickory smoke
- 1 tablespoon pure maple syrup (optional)
- ½ teaspoon smoked paprika
- ¼ teaspoon onion powder
- ¼ teaspoon ground white pepper
- 2 cups unsweetened coconut flakes (not desiccated)

1. Preheat your oven to 350°F (180°C) and line a baking sheet with parchment paper or aluminum foil. Avoid using a silicone mat as the ingredients may stain the surface.
2. In a large bowl, combine the tamari, liquid smoke, optional maple syrup, paprika, onion powder, and ground white pepper. Add the coconut flakes and gently toss until they are thoroughly coated. Allow the mixture to sit for 10 minutes, then stir again before spreading the coconut evenly on the prepared baking sheet. 3. Bake the coconut flakes for 12 minutes until they appear dry and have a golden brown color, avoiding them becoming too dark. 4. Allow the baked coconut flakes to cool completely on the baking sheet. 5. Store the coconut flakes in an airtight container at room temperature for up to 2 weeks, or if desired, freeze them for up to 2 months.

Per Serving: (1 tablespoon)
calories: 36 | fat: 3g | protein: 1g | carbs: 2g | fiber: 1g

Garam Masala

Prep time: 5 minutes | **Cook time:** 0 minutes | **Makes ½ cup**

2 tablespoons black peppercorns	nutmeg or 1¼ teaspoons ground nutmeg
2 tablespoons coriander seeds	1 teaspoon ground cinnamon
2 tablespoons cumin seeds	1 teaspoon whole cloves
1 teaspoon freshly grated	¼ teaspoon cardamom seeds

1. Pulse all the ingredients in a clean coffee grinder until thoroughly combined. Store in an airtight container for up to 6 months.

Per Serving: (½ cup)
calories: 132 | fat: 6g | protein: 5g | carbs: 23g | fiber: 11g

High Protein Black Bean Dip

Prep time: 10 minutes | **Cook time:** 0 minutes | **Serves 3**

4 cups black beans, cooked, rinsed, and drained	1 tablespoon olive oil (optional)
2 tablespoons minced garlic	1 tablespoon lemon juice
2 tablespoons Italian seasoning	¼ teaspoon salt, to taste (optional)
2 tablespoons onion powder	

1. Place black beans in a large bowl and mash them with a fork until everything is mostly smooth. Stir in the remaining ingredients and incorporate thoroughly. The mixture should be smooth and creamy. Add some additional salt (if desired) and lemon juice to taste and serve at room temperature.

Per Serving:
calories: 398 | fat: 7g | protein: 21g | carbs: 63g | fiber: 16g

Tofu Veggie Gravy Bowl

Prep time: 15 minutes | **Cook time:** 10 minutes | **Serves 4**

Gravy:	steamed
6 tablespoons water	1 cup evenly chopped zucchini, steamed
¼ cup diced red, white, or yellow onion	1 cup chopped carrots, steamed
2 tablespoons whole wheat or all-purpose flour	½ (14-ounce / 397-g) block extra-firm tofu, pressed and cut into ½-inch cubes
1 cup vegetable broth	
Veggie Base:	
1 cup evenly sliced broccoli,	

1. In a medium pan over medium heat, heat the water and onion and cook for 3 minutes or until the onion becomes tender and translucent. 2. Reduce the heat to low, add the flour, and stir until your roux has a smooth consistency, 2 to 3 minutes. It should resemble a paste. 3. Add broth and stir over low heat until the gravy thickens, 3 to 4 minutes. 4. On a plate, arrange the broccoli, zucchini, carrots, and tofu, and pour the gravy over this base. Serve immediately.

Per Serving:
calories: 86 | fat: 4g | protein: 7g | carbs: 9g | fiber: 2g

Peanut Butter

Prep time: 15 minutes | **Cook time:** 10 minutes | **Makes 2 cups**

2 cups raw and unsalted peanuts	½ teaspoon sea salt (optional)

1. Preheat your oven to 375ºF (190ºC). 2. Roast the peanuts in the oven for approximately 10 minutes. Once roasted, transfer the peanuts to a food processor and process them for about 1 minute. Don't forget to scrape down the sides of the food processor. If desired, add sea salt and blend again for another minute, repeating until you achieve the desired consistency. 3. For optimal flavor, refrigerate the mixture before serving.

Per Serving:
calories: 153 | fat: 11g | protein: 5g | carbs: 8g | fiber: 1g

Cashew Cheese Spread

Prep time: 5 minutes | **Cook time:** 0 minutes | **Serves 5**

1 cup water	½ teaspoon salt (optional)
1 cup raw cashews	1 teaspoon garlic powder (optional)
1 teaspoon nutritional yeast	

1. In a medium-sized bowl, soak the cashews in water for 6 hours. After soaking, drain the cashews and transfer them to a food processor. Add 1 cup of water and all the other ingredients, then blend until smooth. 2. You can enjoy the mixture right away or store it for later use. For the most delightful flavor, serve it chilled.

Per Serving:
calories: 151 | fat: 11g | protein: 5g | carbs: 9g | fiber: 1g

Nutty Plant-Based Parmesan

Prep time: 10 minutes | **Cook time:** 0 minutes | **Makes 1½ cups**

1 cup raw cashews	½ teaspoon salt (optional)
½ cup nutritional yeast	

1. Using a blender, pulse the cashews until they turn into a fine dust. Transfer the cashew dust to a small bowl and mix it with nutritional yeast and optional salt, thoroughly combining the ingredients using a spoon. For storage, transfer any remaining mixture to an airtight container and keep it refrigerated for up to 10 days or freeze it for up to 3 months.

Per Serving:
calories: 79 | fat: 5g | protein: 3g | carbs: 5g | fiber: 0g

Dulse Rose Za'atar

Prep time: 5 minutes | Cook time: 0 minutes | Makes 6 tablespoons

¼ cup raw unhulled sesame seeds, toasted
2 tablespoons dried organic rose petals
1 tablespoon toasted dulse flakes
1 teaspoon ground sumac
1 teaspoon dried thyme
½ teaspoon flaky sea salt (optional)

1. Combine the sesame seeds, rose petals, dulse, sumac, thyme, and salt, if using, in a small jar or bowl and stir to combine. Store in a tightly sealed jar for up to 3 months.

Per Serving: (1 tablespoon)
calories: 44 | fat: 4g | protein: 1g | carbs: 2g | fiber: 1g

Super-Simple Guacamole

Prep time: 10 minutes | Cook time: 0 minutes | Makes 1½ cups

2 avocados, peeled and pitted
Juice of ½ lime
Pinch of salt (optional)
2 tablespoons chopped fresh cilantro
1 tomato, chopped
1 scallion, white and green parts, chopped

1. In a medium bowl, combine the avocados, lime juice, and salt (if using) and mash together until it reaches your desired consistency. Add the cilantro, tomato, and scallion and mix well. Serve immediately.

Per Serving:
calories: 113 | fat: 10g | protein: 2g | carbs: 7g | fiber: 5g

Miso Gravy

Prep time: 10 minutes | Cook time: 10 minutes | Serves 12

½ cup whole wheat flour
2 garlic cloves, chopped
2½ cups water
½ cup nutritional yeast
3 tablespoons red miso
2 tablespoons apple cider vinegar
2 tablespoons maple syrup (optional)
2 tablespoons tahini
¼ teaspoon black pepper
Salt to taste (optional)

1. Place a medium saucepan over medium heat. Add the flour and garlic. Cook, stirring often, until the garlic is soft and the flour smells toasty, about 3 minutes. 2. Increase the heat to medium-high and add the water, whisking constantly. When the mixture starts to thicken, remove from the heat. (This should take about 3 minutes, and it will be pourable but require the assistance of a spatula.) 3. Use a spatula to transfer the garlic-flour mixture to a blender; add the nutritional yeast, miso, vinegar, maple syrup (if desired), tahini, and pepper. Starting on low and working up to high, blend until thoroughly combined. 4. Taste and adjust seasoning as needed, and serve. The gravy can be refrigerated in an airtight container for up to 4 days.

Per Serving:
calories: 73 | fat: 2g | protein: 5g | carbs: 10g | fiber: 2g

Everyday Pesto

Prep time: 5 minutes | Cook time: 5 minutes | Makes 1 cup

4 cups packed fresh basil leaves
¼ cup raw cashews
2 tablespoons nutritional yeast
1 garlic clove
¼ teaspoon freshly ground black pepper
3 tablespoons boiling water, plus more as needed

1. Mix the basil, cashews, nutritional yeast, garlic, pepper in a food processor, and boiling water until smooth. Add more water to thin until you have a smooth, slightly thick mixture. 2. Refrigerate in a sealed jar for up to 1 month.

Per Serving: (2 tablespoons)
calories: 35 | fat: 2g | protein: 3g | carbs: 2g | fiber: 1g

BBQ Sauce

Prep time: 5 minutes | Cook time: 0 minutes | Serves 16

2 cups canned or fresh tomato cubes
5 pitted dates
3 tablespoons smoked paprika
2 tablespoons garlic powder
2 tablespoons onion powder

1. Combine all the ingredients in a blender or food processor and blend until a smooth sauce forms. 2. Transfer the BBQ sauce to an airtight container and store it in the refrigerator for up to 3 days. Alternatively, you can freeze the sauce for a maximum of 60 days. When needed, simply thaw it at room temperature before using.

Per Serving:
calories: 11 | fat: 0g | protein: 0g | carbs: 2g | fiber: 0g

Simple Berry-Chia Jam

Prep time: 2 minutes | Cook time: 0 minutes | Makes 1½ cups

2 cups frozen organic berries, any variety or a mixture
1 teaspoon fresh lemon juice
2 tablespoons chia seeds
1 to 2 tablespoons date syrup or agave nectar (optional)

1. Use a food processor to pulse the berries until they are well chopped but not fully pureed. 2. Add the lemon juice, chia seeds, and syrup (if using) to the food processor and pulse briefly to combine the ingredients. 3. Transfer the mixture into an airtight jar or container, then refrigerate it overnight to allow the jam to thicken. 4. That's all! Store the jam in the refrigerator for 5 to 7 days.

Per Serving:
calories: 53 | fat: 1g | protein: 1g | carbs: 10g | fiber: 2g

Spicy Italian Vinaigrette

Prep time: 5 minutes | Cook time: 0 minutes | Makes 1 cup

1 cup apple cider vinegar
½ cup extra-virgin olive oil (optional)
2 teaspoons maple syrup (optional)
2 teaspoons Italian seasoning
¼ teaspoon salt (optional)
¼ teaspoon black pepper
½ teaspoon garlic powder
Pinch red pepper flakes

1. Combine the apple cider vinegar, olive oil, maple syrup, Italian seasoning, salt (if using), black pepper, garlic powder, and red pepper flakes in a jar, cover, and shake until well blended. The dressing can be stored in the refrigerator for up to 2 weeks.

Per Serving:
calories: 131 | fat: 14g | protein: 0g | carbs: 2g | fiber: 0g

Roasted Jalapeño and Lime Guacamole

Prep time: 5 minutes | Cook time: 10 minutes | Serves 4

1 to 3 jalapeños
1 avocado, peeled and pitted
1 tablespoon freshly squeezed lime juice

1. Preheat the oven to 400ºF (205ºC). Line a baking sheet with parchment paper. 2. Place the jalapeños on the baking sheet and roast for 8 minutes. (The jalapeño can also be roasted on a grill for 5 minutes, if you already have it fired up.) 3. Slice the jalapeños down the center, and remove the seeds. Then cut the top stem off, and dice into ⅛-inch pieces. Wash your hands immediately after handling the jalapeños. 4. In a medium bowl, use a fork to mash together the avocado, jalapeño pieces, and lime juice. Continue mashing and mixing until the guacamole reaches your preferred consistency, and serve.

Per Serving:
calories: 77 | fat: 7g | protein: 1g | carbs: 5g | fiber: 3g

Roasted Bell Pepper Wedges

Prep time: 5 minutes | Cook time: 25 minutes | Makes 1½ cups

2 large red bell peppers, seeded and cut into wedges
1 tablespoon freshly squeezed lemon juice
Pinch freshly ground black pepper
½ teaspoon garlic powder (optional)
½ teaspoon cumin seeds (optional)

1. Preheat the oven to 425ºF (220ºC). 2. Place the bell pepper wedges in a large mixing bowl; then add the lemon juice, black pepper, garlic powder (if using), and cumin seeds (if using). Toss to combine. 3. Place the bell pepper wedges cut-side down on a baking sheet lined with nonstick foil or parchment paper. 4. Bake for 20 to 25 minutes until soft and lightly charred. Remove from the oven and cool for up to 20 minutes. Store in the refrigerator in an airtight container for up to 5 days.

Per Serving:
calories: 53 | fat: 1g | protein: 2g | carbs: 10g | fiber: 4g

Dreamy Lemon Curd

Prep time: 10 minutes | Cook time: 5 minutes | Makes 1 cup

¼ cup maple syrup or raw agave nectar (optional)
½ cup full-fat coconut milk
⅓ cup fresh lemon juice
¼ cup room temperature coconut oil (optional)
⅛ teaspoon ground turmeric
⅛ teaspoon sea salt (optional)
2 teaspoons lemon zest
2 tablespoons arrowroot powder

1. In a medium saucepan over medium heat, combine the maple syrup, coconut milk, lemon juice, coconut oil, ground tumeric, sea salt, if using, and lemon zest. Bring the mixture to a light boil, whisking occasionally. 2. When some bubbles start to break the surface, add the arrowroot powder to the saucepan, and whisk constantly as the mixture simmers. After the curd has thickened enough to coat the back of a spoon rather thickly, remove from the heat. 3. Quickly scrape the curd into a jar or bowl. Let it cool slightly at room temperature before pressing a piece of plastic wrap onto the surface of the curd. Store the lemon curd in the refrigerator for up to 1 week.

Per Serving: (¼ cup)
calories: 249 | fat: 20g | protein: 1g | carbs: 17g | fiber: 1g

Oat Milk

Prep time: 5 minutes | Cook time: 0 minutes | Makes 4 cups

1 cup rolled oats
3 dates, pitted (optional)
4 cups water

1. In a blender, combine the oats, dates (if using), and water and blend on high for 45 seconds, until the oats are pulverized and the liquid looks creamy. Be careful not to overblend, as the texture will become slimy and unpleasant. 2. Pour the mixture through a nut milk bag, cheesecloth, or fine-mesh sieve to strain out all the small pieces. Pour it into an airtight storage container and chill for up to 4 days.

Per Serving:
calories: 90 | fat: 3g | protein: 1g | carbs: 13g | fiber: 0g

Appendix 1: Measurement Conversion Chart

VOLUME EQUIVALENTS(DRY)

US STANDARD	METRIC (APPROXIMATE)
1/8 teaspoon	0.5 mL
1/4 teaspoon	1 mL
1/2 teaspoon	2 mL
3/4 teaspoon	4 mL
1 teaspoon	5 mL
1 tablespoon	15 mL
1/4 cup	59 mL
1/2 cup	118 mL
3/4 cup	177 mL
1 cup	235 mL
2 cups	475 mL
3 cups	700 mL
4 cups	1 L

WEIGHT EQUIVALENTS

US STANDARD	METRIC (APPROXIMATE)
1 ounce	28 g
2 ounces	57 g
5 ounces	142 g
10 ounces	284 g
15 ounces	425 g
16 ounces (1 pound)	455 g
1.5 pounds	680 g
2 pounds	907 g

VOLUME EQUIVALENTS(LIQUID)

US STANDARD	US STANDARD (OUNCES)	METRIC (APPROXIMATE)
2 tablespoons	1 fl.oz.	30 mL
1/4 cup	2 fl.oz.	60 mL
1/2 cup	4 fl.oz.	120 mL
1 cup	8 fl.oz.	240 mL
1 1/2 cup	12 fl.oz.	355 mL
2 cups or 1 pint	16 fl.oz.	475 mL
4 cups or 1 quart	32 fl.oz.	1 L
1 gallon	128 fl.oz.	4 L

TEMPERATURES EQUIVALENTS

FAHRENHEIT(F)	CELSIUS(C) (APPROXIMATE)
225 °F	107 °C
250 °F	120 °C
275 °F	135 °C
300 °F	150 °C
325 °F	160 °C
350 °F	180 °C
375 °F	190 °C
400 °F	205 °C
425 °F	220 °C
450 °F	235 °C
475 °F	245 °C
500 °F	260 °C

Appendix 2: The Dirty Dozen and Clean Fifteen

The Environmental Working Group (EWG) is a nonprofit, nonpartisan organization dedicated to protecting human health and the environment Its mission is to empower people to live healthier lives in a healthier environment. This organization publishes an annual list of the twelve kinds of produce, in sequence, that have the highest amount of pesticide residue-the Dirty Dozen-as well as a list of the fifteen kinds ofproduce that have the least amount of pesticide residue-the Clean Fifteen.

THE DIRTY DOZEN

- The 2016 Dirty Dozen includes the following produce. These are considered among the year's most important produce to buy organic:

Strawberries	Spinach
Apples	Tomatoes
Nectarines	Bell peppers
Peaches	Cherry tomatoes
Celery	Cucumbers
Grapes	Kale/collard greens
Cherries	Hot peppers

- The Dirty Dozen list contains two additional itemskale/collard greens and hot peppers-because they tend to contain trace levels of highly hazardous pesticides.

THE CLEAN FIFTEEN

- The least critical to buy organically are the Clean Fifteen list. The following are on the 2016 list:

Avocados	Papayas
Corn	Kiw
Pineapples	Eggplant
Cabbage	Honeydew
Sweet peas	Grapefruit
Onions	Cantaloupe
Asparagus	Cauliflower
Mangos	

- Some of the sweet corn sold in the United States are made from genetically engineered (GE) seedstock. Buy organic varieties of these crops to avoid GE produce.

Appendix 3: Recipe Index

A

Adventure Bars	61
Almond and Protein Shake	13
Almond Anise Biscotti	37
Almond-Date Energy Bites	37
Apple Broccoli Crunch Bowl	70
Apple Cinnamon Oats Bowl	18
Apple Crisp	42
Apricot Pistachio Energy Squares	61
Avocado Tartare	50
Avocado Toast	16

B

Baby Potatoes with Dill, Chives, and Garlic	52
Baked Spaghetti Squash with Spicy Lentil Sauce	51
Baked Spaghetti Squash with Swiss Chard	50
Baked Tempeh Nuggets	31
Baked Vegetable Chips	59
Banana Soft Serve	38
Banana, Date and Coconut Muesli	14
Barley and White Bean Pilaf	31
Basil Pesto	92
BBQ Sauce	96
Bean and Mushroom Chili	87
Best Whole Wheat Pancakes	15
Better-Than-Mom's Banana Bread	37
Black Sesame–Ginger Quick Bread	44
Blackened Sprouts	52
Blueberry and Peanut Butter Parfait Bowls	14
Blueberry Muffin Loaf	40
Blueberry-Lime Sorbet	39
Bowl	74
Breakfast Hummus on Toast	16
Broccoli and "Cheddar" Soup	85
Broccoli Caesar with Smoky Tempeh Bits	71
Broccolini on Fire	53
Brown Lentil Stew with Avocado Salsa	87
Buckwheat Sesame Milk	25
Bulgur Chickpea Pilaf	33
Bulgur, Cucumber and Tomato Salad	72

C

Cabbage Salad and Peanut Butter Vinaigrette	67
Caramel-Coconut Frosted Brownies	38
Caramelized Onion Potato Salad	74
Caribbean Coconut Collards and Sweet Potatoes	81
Carrot Ginger Soup	77
Cashew Cheese Spread	95
Cauliflower Bake Topping	89
Cauliflower Béchamel	21
Cauliflower Scramble	17
Chana Saag	32
Cheesy Sprinkle	22
Cherry Chocolate Bark	39
Cherry Chocolate Hemp Balls	60
Cherry Pecan Granola Bars	12
Chickpea Cookie Dough	63
Chickpea Pâté	28
Chickpea Tortilla Fajita Stack	30
Chilean Bean Stew	83
Chipotle Black Bean Soup	82
Chocolate Pudding with Raspberries and Mint	40
Chocolate-Covered Strawberries	40
Chorizo Chickpea Bowl	29
Cilantro-Coconut Pesto	91
Cleansing Morning Lemonade	18
Coconut "Bacon" Bits	94
Coconut Chia Pudding	42
Coconut Crumble Bars	44
Coconut Curry Soup	83
Coconut Watercress Soup	78
Creamy Avocado-Lime Dressing	23
Creamy Balsamic Dressing	90
Creamy Mushroom Gravy	94
Creamy Nut Sauce	89
Croutons	24
Cumin-Citrus Roasted Carrots	51
Curried Zucchini Soup	81

D

"Don't Waste the Good Stuff" Squash Soup	79
Dreamy Lemon Curd	97
Dulse Rose Za'atar	96

E

Eggplant and Chickpea Rice Pilaf	35
Eggplant Bacon	18

Everyday Pesto · 96

F

Fancy Instant Ramen Soup · 82
Fancy Rice · 33
Farro Tabbouleh · 34
Fava Bean Salad · 69
Fennel and Cherry Tomato Gratin · 48
Fermented Carrots with Turmeric and Ginger · 52
Fiery Couscous Salad · 73
Forbidden Black Rice and Edamame Salad · 72
Fresh Tomato Salsa · 26
Fried Rice with Tofu Scramble · 31
Fruit Salad with Zesty Citrus Couscous · 15
Ful Medames (Egyptian Breakfast Beans) · 17
Ful Nabed (Egyptian Fava Bean Soup) · 77

G

Garam Masala · 95
Garlic Hummus · 60
Garlic Mashed Potatoes · 46
Garlicky Winter Vegetable and White Bean Mash · 51
Gluten-Free Vegan Waffles · 43
Golden Split Pea Soup · 80
Gooey Bittersweet Chocolate Pudding Cake · 41
Grain-Free Porridge · 15
Greek Salad in a Jar · 71
Green Mix Salad · 68
Green Split Peas · 21
Greener Guacamole · 25
Guacamole · 64
Gut-Healing Sauerkraut · 22

H

Harissa · 94
Hearty Veggie Hoagies · 34
Hemp Mylk · 24
Herbed Millet Pizza Crust · 21
High Protein Black Bean Dip · 95
High-Protein Chocolate Blender Muffins · 19

I

Italian Lentil Soup · 80

J

Jicama-Citrus Pickle · 53

K

Kalamata Olives and White Bean Dip · 90
Kale and Lentil Stew · 84
Kale White Bean Soup · 84
Kale, Black Bean and Quinoa Salad · 67

Kasha Varnishkes (Buckwheat Groats with Bow-Tie Pasta) · 34
Korean Tahini BBQ Sauce · 91

L

Leaf and Stem Green Tortilla Soup · 86
Lemon Mint Tahini Cream · 90
Lemon-Pepper Bean Dip with Rosemary · 64
Lemon-Thyme Dressing · 25
Lemony Steamed Kale with Olives · 52
Lentil Chili · 86
Lentil Rice Soup · 84
Lentil Salad with Lemon and Fresh Herbs · 74
Lentil Soup · 80
Lentil Soup with Cauliflower, Potatoes and Spinach · 82
Lentil-Mushroom No-Meat Pasta (Bolognese) · 30
Lentil, Lemon and Mushroom Salad · 70
Lima Bean Stew · 84
Lime-Mint Soup · 85
Loaded Sweet Apple "Nachos" · 58
Lucky Black-Eyed Pea Stew · 28

M

Mac 'N' Mince · 33
Maca-Mint Smoothie · 11
Mama Mia Marinara Sauce · 25
Mango Ginger Kombucha Mimosas · 11
Mango Lentil Salad · 68
Mango Plantain Nice Cream · 57
Mango Satay Tempeh Bowl · 29
Mango Sticky Rice · 41
Mango-Orange Dressing · 24
Maple-Dijon Dressing · 24
Maple-Spice Buckwheat Crispies Cereal · 14
Maple, Apple, and Walnut Great Grains · 11
Mexican Quinoa Bowl · 34
Mexikale Crisps · 58
Mild Harissa Sauce · 90
Millet Porridge · 17
Minestrone · 77
15-Minute French Fries · 63
20-Minute Cashew Cheese Sauce · 23
Miso Gravy · 96
Miso Noodle Soup with Shiitake Mushrooms · 78
Miso Nori Chips · 62
Mixed Beans Chili · 32
Mocha Chocolate Brownie Bars · 65
Mock Tuna Salad · 67
Mujadara (Lentils with Rice and Caramelized Onions) · 33

N

Nacho Cheese · 65
Nice Cream · 40
Nilla Cookies · 43
No-Bake Cereal Date Bars · 59

No-Bake Mocha Cheesecake · 41
Nori Snack Rolls · 65
North African Chickpeas and Vegetables · 32
Not-So-Fat Guacamole · 24
Nut or Seed Butter · 89
Nut-Crusted Tofu · 29
Nutty Plant-Based Parmesan · 95

O

Oat Crunch Apple Crisp · 57
Oat Milk · 97
Oil-Free Hummus · 25
Oil-Free Sundried Tomato and Oregano Dressing · 89
Orange Cranberry Power Cookies · 56
Orzo "Risotto" · 30
Overnight Muesli · 16
Overnight Pumpkin Spice Chia Pudding · 12

P

Pan con Tomate · 11
Paradise Island Overnight Oatmeal · 18
Pasta Marinara with Spicy Italian Bean Balls · 35
Peanut Butter · 95
Peanut Butter Apple Sauce · 90
Peanut Butter Balls · 61
Peanut Butter Chocolate Bars · 63
Peanut Butter Chocolate Seed Balls · 57
Peanut Butter Nice Cream · 42
Peanut Butter Snack Squares · 58
Peanut Milk · 25
Perfect Marinara Sauce · 92
Pico de Gallo · 93
Pineapple Chutney · 21
Plant-Based Fish Sauce · 23
Plant-Powered "Sour Cream" · 92
Popeye Protein Balls · 62
Potato and Veggie Breakfast Casserole · 11
Potato, Carrot, and Mushroom Stew · 78
Potato, Corn and Bean Soup · 79
Powerhouse Protein Shake · 12
Pressure Cooker Tender Patties · 64
Protein Peanut Butter Balls · 56
Provencal Beans and Tomato Salad · 72
Pump Up the Power Energy Balls · 59
Pumpkin Bread Pudding · 38
Pumpkin Spice Bread · 39
Pure Nut Mylk · 24

Q

Quick and Easy Thai Vegetable Stew · 81
Quick Bean Sauce · 94
Quick Mole Sauce · 93
Quick Spelt Bread · 93
Quinoa · 22

Quinoa Arugula Salad · 68
Quinoa Primavera · 28

R

Ratatouille · 48
Raw Date Chocolate Balls · 65
Red Flannel Beet Hash with Dill · 17
Red Lentil Dal · 31
Red Lentil Pâté · 28
Refrigerator Pickles · 91
Roasted Balsamic Beets · 54
Roasted Bell Pepper Wedges · 97
Roasted Jalapeño and Lime Guacamole · 97
Roasted Potato and Cauliflower Soup · 85
Roasted Red Pepper and Butternut Squash Soup · 80
Roasted Root Vegetable Hash · 13
Roasted Root Vegetable Salad Bulgur Lettuce Cups · 75
Roasted Vegetable and Lentil Salad · 73
Romesco-Style Hummus · 64

S

Salsa Verde · 23
Sautéed Root Vegetables with Parsley, Poppy Seeds, and Lemon · 47
Savory Quinoa Breakfast Cups · 13
Savory Roasted Chickpeas · 56
Savory Sweet Potato Casserole · 46
Sesame-Tamari Portable Rice Balls · 58
Sheet-Pan Garlicky Kale · 48
Shiitake Bakin' · 19
Showtime Popcorn · 60
Sick Day Soup · 78
Simple Berry-Chia Jam · 96
Skillet Cauliflower Bites · 62
Slow Cooker Chipotle Tacos · 56
Slow Cooker Versatile Seitan Balls · 62
Small-Batch Roasted Soup · 82
Smoky Mushrooms · 91
Smoky Saffron Chickpea, Chard, and Rice Soup · 85
Sour Cream · 92
Southwest Stuffed Peppers · 35
Spaghetti Squash with Marinara and Veggies · 93
Spanish Chickpea Stew · 83
Spelt Berry Hot Breakfast Cereal · 16
Spiced Kidney Bean Curry · 35
Spiced Sorghum and Berries · 15
Spicy Black Bean Dip · 61
Spicy Butternut Squash Bisque · 47
Spicy Cilantro Pesto · 21
Spicy Italian Vinaigrette · 97
Spicy Miso-Roasted Tomatoes and Eggplant · 53
Spinach Salad with Sweet Smoky Dressing · 70
Split Pea Soup · 86
Spring All-Purpose Seasoning · 90
Spring Breakfast Salad · 18
Spring Steamed Vegetables with Savory Goji Berry Cream · 49

Steamed Kabocha Squash with Nori and Scallions ··· 53
Stir-Fried Vegetables with Miso and Sake ··· 47
Stone Fruit Chia Pudding ··· 43
Strawberry Dressing ··· 26
Strawberry-Pistachio Salad ··· 69
Succotash Salad ··· 68
Sunshine Everything Crackers ··· 57
Sunshine Muffins ··· 14
Super-Simple Guacamole ··· 96
Superfood Caramels ··· 42
Sweet Potato and Black Bean Quesadillas ··· 60
Sweet Potato and Chocolate Pudding ··· 43
Sweet Potato Toasts with Avocado Mash and Tahini ··· 13

T

Tahini Dressing ··· 22
Tahini Green Beans ··· 29
Tandoori-Rubbed Portobellos with Cool Cilantro Sauce ··· 50
Tea Scones ··· 39
Tempeh Bacon ··· 23
Tempeh Breakfast Sausage ··· 12
Teriyaki Mushrooms ··· 47
Toast Points ··· 60
Tofu and Zoodles Dinner Salad ··· 73
Tofu Sour Cream ··· 26
Tofu Veggie Gravy Bowl ··· 95
Tomato Sauce ··· 22
Tomato, Corn and Bean Salad ··· 69
Tortilla Chips ··· 61
Tuscan Bean Stew ··· 77
Tuscan White Bean Salad ··· 67
Two-Minute Turtles ··· 41

U

Ultimate Veggie Wrap with Kale Pesto ··· 49

V

Vanilla Almond Date Balls ··· 65
Vanilla Bean Whip ··· 37
Vanilla Buckwheat Porridge ··· 19
Vanilla Protein Pancakes ··· 16
Vanilla-Cinnamon Fruit Cocktail ··· 64
Vegan "Toona" Salad ··· 71
Vegan Goulash ··· 48
Vegetable Spring Rolls with Spicy Peanut Dipping Sauce ··· 49
Veggie Chow Mein ··· 91

W

Warm Lentil Salad ··· 69
Warm Maple Protein Oatmeal ··· 12
Warm Sweet Potato and Brussels Sprout Salad ··· 68
Watermelon with Coconut-Lime Yogurt ··· 56
Weeknight Root Vegetable Dhal ··· 79
Whipped Lentil Chipotle Dip ··· 92
White Bean Caponata ··· 59
White Bean Tzatziki Dip ··· 63
White Bean, Butternut Squash, and Kale Soup ··· 81
White Beans Summer Salad ··· 72
Winter Squash Soup ··· 83

Y

Yellow Bell Pepper Boats ··· 46

Z

Zesty Orange-Cranberry Energy Bites ··· 38
Zucchini "Parmesan" ··· 46
Zucchini Bread Oatmeal ··· 19

Made in United States
Orlando, FL
27 July 2024